The Doctor's Guide
to You
and Your Colon

THE DOCTOR'S GUIDE TO YOU AND YOUR COLON

by Martin E. Plaut, M.D.

Illustrations by Tom Toles

HARPER & ROW, PUBLISHERS, New York
Cambridge, Philadelphia, San Francisco,
London, Mexico City, São Paulo, Sydney

1817

This book is for A.P.

THE DOCTOR'S GUIDE TO YOU AND YOUR COLON. Copyright © 1982 by Martin E. Plaut, M.D. All rights reserved. Printed in the United States of America. No part of this book may be used or reproduced in any manner whatsoever without written permission except in the case of brief quotations embodied in critical articles and reviews. For information address Harper & Row, Publishers, Inc., 10 East 53rd Street, New York, N.Y. 10022. Published simultaneously in Canada by Fitzhenry & Whiteside Limited, Toronto.

FIRST EDITION

Library of Congress Cataloging in Publication Data

The doctor's guide to you and your colon.
Includes index.
1. Colon (Anatomy)—Diseases. 2. Hemorrhoids.
I. Title.
RC860.M36   1982   616.3′4   80-7861
ISBN 0-06-014948-5   AACR2

82 83 84 85 86 10 9 8 7 6 5 4 3 2 1

Contents

Acknowledgments

Major contributors to this book include the following experts in medicine, gastroenterology, and infectious disease: Andrew G. Plaut, M.D.: Three Serious Diseases of the Colon, and Hemorrhoids; David J. Kudzma, M.D.: How the Bowel Works; Michael D. Levitt, M.D.: Gas; Alan I. Leibowitz, M.D.: Fiber; Gerald S. Keusch, M.D. and Sherwood L. Gorbach, M.D.: *Turista*.

I also thank those who offered helpful suggestions: Drs. Milton Weiser, Richard Lee; Nancy Tobin Willig, and Jeff Simon. Tom Toles, editorial cartoonist for the Buffalo *Courier-Express*, provided drawings that show his unique talent. Leanne Scheira was a valued editorial assistant.

Last, as a writer, I am grateful to B.R., whose enthusiasm for my manuscript allowed me to sprint out of the starting gate, and N.C., who kept me from going out on the turns.   —Martin E. Plaut, M.D.

The purpose of this book is to make you aware of the normal functioning of the colon and how it can go awry. The assessment of symptoms requires an expert. Proper diagnosis and therapy of all illnesses of the bowel, real or apparent, call for careful attention to your complaints by your doctor.

1
Introduction

A reliable set of bowels is worth more to a man than any quantity of brains.

Josh Billings
(Henry Wheeler Shaw)

Had this statement been uttered by an aging Englishman sipping his gin and tonic on some shaded veranda in India in the twenties, we could have gained insight into the reason for the subsequent loss of England's empire. As part of the monologue on a late-night television show, the comment would cause genuine laughter in the audience and evoke grunts of delight from forty million viewers. A psychiatrist who heard a patient speak these words would at least look up from his own folded hands.

Most preoccupations fade or intensify, but for millions of people who worry about "the bowels" (actually, the colon), the concern remains steadfast. Many doctors are convinced that bowel and bowel-related complaints are more common than any other single health complaint that prompts patients to visit their offices. The facts support this impression. A worldwide marketing research firm collected data on symptoms that brought adult patients in America to the offices of private physicians during the year 1980. *The symptom of abdominal pain was reported more often than even back pain or headache.*

Moreover, an unknown but obviously large number of additional people sought relief from constipation, abdominal pain, gas, diarrhea, or hemorrhoids in other health-care facilities, including hospital emergency rooms, outpatient departments of hospitals, and employee health clinics. And even this large number of people with bowel complaints omits those who sought advice—and usually medicine—from their neighborhood pharmacist.

Surveys of drugs purchased over the counter also understate the scope and extent of bowel complaints in American adults. For every adult who purchases a laxative or an antacid in a pharmacy, someone else does the same in a supermarket. Forty million Americans use laxatives, and eight million of these are "heavy" users, at least once a week. Antacids are swallowed by ulcer patients, to be sure, but also by those whose "nervous stomachs" are really expressions of gastroenteritis, excess intestinal gas, or the disordered intestinal motion that many call "spastic colon." All new medical interns quickly learn that patients hospitalized for nearly any illness will invariably require three kinds of medicine: something for pain relief, something to aid sleep, and something for the bowel.

Unfortunately, in our society many prefer to laugh off problems of the bowel, rather than discuss them in a serious, straightforward fashion. Comedy routines based upon, say, respiration and coughing are unknown to us, and the incredibly complex activities of the nervous system, from simple reflexes to abstract thought, seem to concern us only when age, drugs, or alcohol renders us forgetful, stoned, or uninhibited. Our kidneys maintain salt and water balance by elegant mechanisms that interest only scientists and patients with kidney disease. On the subject of urine, young male writers comment about the height of the arc, and older ones stress the sense of relief. Ordinary citizens have no interest in their lymph nodes, livers, and spleens; and organs as diverse as pituitary and thymus glands function unseen and ignored. But present a comedy sketch wherein a Russian cosmonaut reports to earth that he's encountered "kaka" as he walks on the moon, and a Las Vegas casino will sign up the actor and pay him many thousands of dollars to tell the joke twice a night.

Another problem is illustrated by the one-minute dramas played out in endless variation on television, where headache and irritability the night before are followed the next morning by the evacuation of a normal stool and an apparent transformation of personality. The magic was wrought by swallowing a product that resembled chocolate, gum, mints, cream, or mucilage. These commercials sound the message that a day without a bowel movement just won't be the kind of day it *could* be if only regularity were achieved.

The idea that a regular bowel habit means one, only one, but definitely one bowel movement a day is but a single misconception of many concerning the colon and its product discussed in this book. Doctors are consulted every day by otherwise healthy people terribly worried about symptoms described as constipation, diarrhea, or irregularity. Even if a complete medical exam reveals no abnormality of the gastrointestinal tract or any other organ, the worries often persist. Some people complain of alternating periods of constipation and diarrhea, whereas others have problems with gas, abdominal pain, hemorrhoids, or apparent maldigestion. The last complaint concerns stools that float instead of sink, that are bulkier, more odorous, thinner, fatter, more pebbly, less colorful, or softer than "they ought to be."

For millions, the condition of the large bowel and its product can sometimes seem to be of greater concern than the rigors of a job or even the affairs of the world's men and women that some call civilization. When a doctor, in asking a long list of questions about various systems of the body, inquires as to the state of the bowels, some patients blush and say nothing, while others begin an impassioned monologue.

The universal interest in the bowels has to do primarily with the colon or large bowel, and not the stomach and small bowel, where digestion takes place. The colon is a drying tank unrelated to digestion, as doctors know. Yet physicians are at least as bowel conscious as the rest of mankind. A group of gastroenterologists on their way to Mexico City for an international congress a few years ago assumed that some of them would develop *turista* or traveler's diarrhea. In an exercise best labeled an orgy of narcissism, physicians and their families sent appropriately packaged rectal swabs through the mails to the Center for Disease Control in Atlanta, Georgia, both before leaving for Mexico City and upon their return. They dutifully provided samples of stool for exhaustive study when diarrhea struck, as it did for about 40 percent of the adults and children making the journey. A questionnaire about bowel symptoms was also completed. The result of this investigation expanded our knowledge about *turista* and reinforced the notion that doctors, too, are not immune to such problems, and are in need of more information to help control bowel malfunctions.

The purpose of this book is to present this much-needed information, including how the bowel works, then why things *seem* to go wrong when no disease is present, why such conditions as gas, hemorrhoids, or traveler's diarrhea occur, and what can be done to manage or prevent these conditions. Chapter 4, Laxatives, Enemas, and Fiber, discusses these three ways to establish a "regular" bowel habit and the benefit and risks of each approach. Serious diseases *do* afflict the colon, and a chapter on diverticulitis, ulcerative colitis, and cancer of the colon describes these three important diseases in depth. An index allows the reader to look up specific subjects or popular topics of concern, such as the controversy on the value of more fiber in the diet, management of the "spastic" colon, useful treatment of hemorrhoids, the facts about belching, bloating, and flatus, and the difference between diverticulosis and diverticulitis.

This book provides facts about common conditions affecting the bowel, and presents advice on how to manage these problems, yet it is not meant to be a guide to the treatment of bowel disease. We can discuss the management of colon polyps, for example, but you had best discuss the problem of *your* polyp with your physician.

It is not too much to hope that the information presented here will reassure most readers and improve the health of some. This is particularly true for those who worry that simple hemorrhoids will surely require surgery (most will not); that habitual use of laxatives and enemas are inconvenient but not dangerous to health (they can be); or that long-standing variations in bowel habit, especially if accompanied by bloating or vague abdominal pains, require consulting one doctor after another until the correct diagnosis and treatment are determined. Although some persons do, unfortunately, have serious or progressive disease of the bowel, which can necessitate in-depth consultation with several specialists, most do not. We try to indicate which bowel complaints arise in healthy people without bowel disease (such as gas, brief pain with fluctuations in the frequency of bowel habit, a few days without a bowel movement), as well as those that require prompt diagnosis, such as rectal bleeding of *any* amount, even if hemorrhoids are known to exist.

A number of physicians have contributed important ideas to the various chapters of this book, and their names appear elsewhere. As in all areas of medicine, the causes and management of many bowel conditions are still debated. Where opposing views exist, we try to present fairly the present state of our knowledge, or, for example, in considering the cause of ulcerative colitis or cancer of the colon, our relative ignorance.

Now it is time to begin, seated, with perhaps a faint sense of urgency, and yes, even anticipation.

2
How the Bowel Works

A proper bowel movement is a minor blessing. Of course, other personal habits make us feel good, from the tingling smoothness of teeth and gums well-brushed to soft, clean hair recently shampooed. Passing urine too can be a source of impressive relief, depending on how long one has had to wait. Yet the ritual of painlessly moving the bowels provides the kind of special satisfaction that comes with something truly *done*. Many sympathetic doctors, especially gastroenterologists, express the view that a regular bowel habit results from taking bowel function for granted. This is precisely what millions of people preoccupied with "the bowels" cannot do. The process of digesting foodstuffs and eliminating the waste is a complex and fascinating internal event. This chapter presents information about how the bowel works so that we can accept both the action and end product of this organ with the matter-of-factness we have about our hearts or our brains.

The human intestinal tract possesses intricate mechanisms of genuine virtuosity designed to nourish every cell in the human body. Each inch of this curled forty-foot organ system deals masterfully with what arrives from above and passes to regions below. Keep in mind that the human gastrointestinal tract goes from the lips and mouth to the throat and esophagus, then to the stomach, to the small intestine, and then to the colon (large intestine), to end at the rectum and anus. A look at the accompanying illustration shows the small bowel as the narrower loops surrounded by the large bowel, starting at the cecum and describing almost a rectangle until the loop curves down to the rectum and anus.

The stomach, small bowel, and large bowel demonstrate meal after meal that Nature needn't be beautiful to be admirable. In fact, the proper function of the entire gastrointestinal tract can be described as a process of alchemy in reverse, since delicious food is transformed to an unpleasant-smelling waste product. Yet, as the result of this alchemy, the gastrointestinal tract is able to extract from what we eat and drink the nutrients needed to initiate and maintain the life of each human cell. Every natural process should lead to so ennobling a result!

The complex business of digestion and elimination

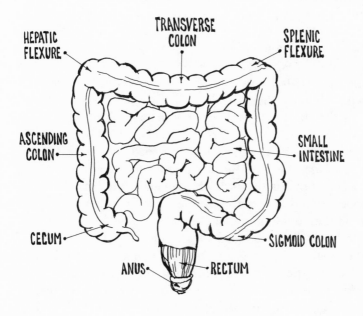

commences at the very top—in the mouth, where the gastrointestinal tract begins. For, even as we chew our daily buttered bread, enzymes in saliva break up the starches present in food. The chewing process also triggers the release in the stomach of both hydrochloric acid and the enzyme called pepsin. This acid and burning brew is crucial for digestion, and awaits each chewed mouthful that passes down the esophagus and enters the rhythmic churn of the stomach.

Even the simple act of swallowing requires complex muscular actions controlled by nerves in the brain that help the esophagus propel food in the right direction. To eat food without trouble while lying down requires that the muscles in the wall of the esophagus correct for changes in position so that food that enters the stomach won't regurgitate or reflux back. The esophagus must also accommodate different-sized swallows of air, liquids, and solids, sometimes in rapidly changing form, as gas bubbles out of soda pop or hard ice cream melts. All these actions and controls require more than a simple connection between mouth and stomach.

People who view television ads for antacids develop the idea that the stomach is a kind of rigid container in which liquids change color when good medicine neutralizes the ill effects of hydrochloric acid. The stomach, in fact, is a muscular churn whose lining cells release the acid necessary for digestion. No food, chewed or not, is truly digested until the life-giving nutrients in it are absorbed through the wall of the small intestine. Digestion first requires that both enzymes and acid chemically chop food thoroughly and completely, much as a Cuisinart does mechanically to a head of lettuce. This task completed, the contents of the stomach now enter the first part of the small intestine through a muscular structure called the *pylorus*. The Greek work *pylorus* means "gatekeeper," but what signals the pyloric gates to open is still not well understood. Once food passes the pylorus it does not, in

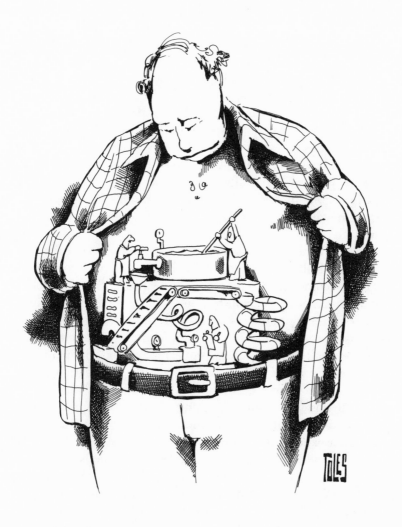

health, back up into the stomach again, even if one lies flat for a nap after a heavy meal. Everything in the normal gastrointestinal tract moves in but one direction.

The main event in the small bowel is digestion. The *duodenum,* so called because of its twelve-inch length, comprises only the first foot of the thirty-five feet of *small* bowel, yet its wall contains openings through which pour some of the most powerful digestive and solubilizing agents known, arriving in the duodenum from the gall bladder and pancreas. These liquids attack the acidified stream of food early in its slow trip, and for good reason. In this process, fats are disintegrated, proteins split, and starches broken into simple sugars. The salts in food crucial to survival, especially sodium and potassium, are also extracted in the small bowel, and vitamins, a variety of trace metals, and water itself are absorbed into the body as well.

Textbooks of a thousand pages or more are needed to describe fully what happens in the small bowel, and the story becomes more complex as research scientists report new findings every month. Some of the elements in the story serve to impress us again with the balancing mechanisms correctly built into every human gut. The contents of the small bowel must be properly liquefied, maintained at a precise pH of acid or base depending on location, and move at the right speed to allow for removal of nutrients. Yet all this would mean nothing without the appearance of bile acids and salts, enzymes, and hormones from the pancreas and gall bladder in exact amounts at just the right moments. For these substances carry out the fracturing and dismantling of the foods we consume in complex forms. Digestion "into" the body requires that food be broken down to simpler molecules, especially since we eat amino acids as beef; fat as incredibly long-chained acids in butter and cream; and carbohydrates as breads and pastries. These foods taste delicious and eating adds enormously to the pleasures of life—in fact, to some, eating

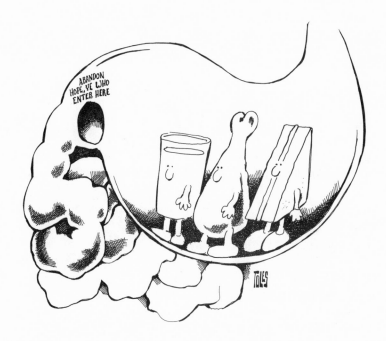

becomes *the* pleasure in life. That simple foods are more easily digested is a general but not invariable truth.

Given the complex nature of digestive processes, it is remarkable that all healthy small bowels work with virtually uniform efficiency. The small bowel has no appetite—it simply does its duty, the level of activity depending on the appetite of its owner. Obese people are not fat because their small bowels more completely absorb food, but because more food has passed their lips. Everything nutritionally useful and digestible is absorbed. What the healthy bowel rejects and sends on down is simply what can't be digested, whether fiber or peach pits.

In striking contrast to the intensity and near frenzy that mark the small intestine's effort, the large bowel (from now on usually called the *colon*) works with comparative torpor. The colon is simply a drying tank four to six feet long. A look at the illustration on page 7 shows the colon facing outward with both small intestine and colon exposed. The appendix is a small curl at the lower left and then comes the cecum, so called because without an opening to the outside it was termed "blind" by the ancient namers of organ parts. The watery fluid that leaves the small bowel enters the cecum and is dried as it journeys up, across, and down (ascending colon, transverse, and descending—the names *do* make sense) through the sigmoid colon and then into the rectum. The trip around the colon—both the twenty-four hours it takes and the four to six feet traversed—allows for time and space so that water present can be reabsorbed into the body. Keep in mind, though, that digestion is virtually complete even before the colon begins to work. This explains why patients who undergo total removal of the colon (the large bowel, remember) can live in perfect health as long as they drink a little more water than others do. The daylong journey through the colon ends as the now largely dehydrated mass of feces fills the rectum as a solid column that asks, then insists on being let out.

The Stool Itself

Color. For over two thousand years, even before Hippocrates's rudimentary experiments to learn about digestion, doctors wondered why stool looks and smells as it does, and what changes in appearance signify in terms of health and disease. Feces are comprised of well-kneaded lumps of undigested food fibers mixed thoroughly with hundreds of billions of germs—bacteria—that normally live in our colons. The other ingredient is water, usually enough to allow for softness yet not so much as to cause diarrhea. Without water the feces become hard, as often occurs in the elderly, those who fail to drink enough water, and people given or taking strong narcotics. Minor additional components of feces may include aged cells that drift off the lining of both the small intestine and colon, intact seeds, and the odd gallstone, tooth fragment, peanut, and bit of thread.

The product is brown because the bacteria living in the colon make brown pigments out of bile acids and salts, chemicals originally present in the bile that flowed into the small intestine to play an important part in digestion. With digestion complete, the brown pigments that remain become part of the wastes moving slowly toward disposal. The exact hue of the fecal brown may vary subtly from day to day and is generally of no importance, but dramatic color changes are always worth noticing. Your feces may appear reddish if you eat beets, turn black if you take iron tablets or bleed from the small intestine, and become nearly white if the fat in the diet is not being digested. Some stools are not whitish yet emerge fat and greasy, and suggest either that mineral oil was used as a laxative, or that a malfunction exists somewhere in the small intestine so that fat is not being absorbed. Greasy stools and weight loss suggest malabsorption and require investigation.

If you are *not* taking iron tablets and have a jet-black stool, it suggests bleeding somewhere in the small intestine. If this occurs, see a doctor without delay. Bright red blood in the stool or on toilet paper represents another warning flag that should never be ignored. Although bleeding hemorrhoids commonly cause red blood to appear on either the feces or the toilet paper, that diagnosis should not be made until a thorough examination in a doctor's office is complete. Even if you *have* bleeding hemorrhoids, as the chapter on that subject makes clear, the rectal bleeding may result from other serious causes, including cancer.

Odor and bacteria. Feces smell as they do because of malodorous gases produced by bacteria that live in the bowel. The chapters on gas and *turista* describe the various kinds of bacteria that reside in the colon and what they are doing there. The lower part of the small bowel and the entire colon house hundreds of billions of tiny bacteria of many different species, and each cherry-sized lump of stool contains countless numbers of these microscopic germs, multiplying freely in the warm, airless recesses of the colon. Most species of bacteria are actually *selected* to grow in the colon by the conditions present, especially the lack of oxygen. These bacteria work on undigested fibers and sugars to form gas. Although the principal objective in passing feces is simply one of elimination, the bacteria residing in the colon and the role of these bacteria in the maintenance of human health are complex subjects actively being investigated. It may offer reassurance to the fastidious to comment here that animals raised with sterile colons, fed sterile food and water, and housed in a germ-free environment will pass stools devoid of bacteria, yet such animals live shorter and less healthy lives than do their litter mates allowed to develop the usual colon flora of bacteria.

Ever since the invention of the microscope we have known that the "wee beasties" of bacteria live in profusion in the colon and pass in the stool. About the turn of the century a Nobel-laureate scientist named Elie Metchnikoff believed that longevity in some eastern Europeans resulted from their eating cheese and yogurt from goat's milk full of bacteria called lactobacilli. We now know that the lactobacilli in yogurt are usually incapable of taking up residence in the human colon, where hundreds of strains of bacteria continuously compete for space, food, and the very right to survive. The relatively few lactobacilli usually pass on through. You may well feel better eating yogurt, as "health"-food stores are fond of predicting, but there's nothing inherently good or even healthy about the bacteria that produce this popular product.

Since a multitude of bacteria are always present in even the smallest lump of feces, the search for the disease-producing bacteria in a person with sudden diarrhea is usually fruitless. Diarrhea can result from an infection of the lining of the small bowel or the colon as a result of viruses, parasites, or bacteria such as *Salmonella* or *Shigella*, as well as from stress or milk (lactose) intolerance, or as a side effect of many medicines such as antibiotics that irritate the bowel wall. With each cause, the abnormality in the colon is that the contents move along too rapidly. Recall that the colon is the site for removal of water from stool. When irritated, as with infection, the colon hurries along what it receives from the small bowel. The drying process is thus incomplete, and watery diarrhea results.

Motion. When diarrhea does not exist, the contents of the colon thicken into a more and more dense mass, are nudged along by a kneading motion of the colon wall, and finally settle as feces in the rectum. Feces normally remain moist, since small amounts of water and bile acids are still present even after the journey through the colon is finished. The bile acids induce the lining of the colon to secrete just a bit of salt and water when the contents become excessively dry. It's impressive how even such a routine task as drying has a built-in physiological control mechanism. Such control of the drying process is crucial or else stool becomes too hard ever to pass painlessly. Older people or those who drink too little water therefore commonly complain of painful constipation.

For a normal bowel movement to occur, the key event is movement. The muscular colon exhibits several kinds of motion, one a constant churning type that keeps the fecal contents close to the bowel wall and allows for removal of water. Another is the squeezing and yielding motion that transports the contents up, across, and down toward the rectum and anus. Third is the vigorous push that usually occurs only once or twice a day and opens the round muscle of the anus. *This remarkable system works automatically and consistently and cannot be aided by pressure on the abdomen or other strenuous efforts to force out the contents during defecation.* If strenuous voluntary efforts were successful, imagine what would happen when we laugh, lift weights, or engage in other kinds of strenuous activity. It is the *internal* motion of the muscular bowel wall, not pressure on the abdomen, that evacuates feces from the bowel. If you suffer from constipation, no attempt to drive out feces by squeezing down will be effective. Many of the world's people, especially in the Orient and Southeast Asia, defecate while squatting instead of sitting, but even this maneuver is designed not so much to exert pressure as to straighten the rectum and lower colon to aid in emptying.

Regularity

Regularity is best thought of as your usual bowel habit. How often should "normal" bowels move? The range of normal varies from three movements a day to one every two weeks. A confidential survey of a hundred thousand adults might uncover the fact that the average person has seven bowel movements per week, or one a day. But to have two bowel movements a day, or one bowel movement every three days for most of one's lifetime is perfectly within the range of normal for some of us. The same can be said of body temperatures of 97° versus 98° F., of heart rates per minute of 60 or 90, or an ideal body weight of 40 kg to 100 kg. For most humans, defecation occurs about once a day, usually in the morning. When the major contraction signaling defecation commences and a toilet is unavailable, the conscious adult holds it in, the muscular contraction subsides, and the urge to defecate ceases. This favorable outcome is due entirely to the holding action of the anal muscle. If the normal "call to stool" goes unheeded and everything quiets down, the major contraction may begin again in a half hour or an hour or, in many people, an entire twenty-four hours will elapse before the urge to defecate again occurs. No harm results if one to ten days pass without a normal bowel movement.

The events that provoke the colon to empty itself are harder to explain scientifically than are the variation and frequency of normal bowel movements. Anxiety, whether before an exam, a speech, or an unpleasant encounter, can set up a substantial contraction of the rectum. Thoroughbred racehorses walking to the starting gate and animals being herded onto vehicles clearly experience the same reaction. The bowel and brain are obviously connected by elaborate and nervous pathways—some still unexplored—that transmit information in both directions. Many of these interactions are well known but only dimly understood. We recognize that emotions "get our bowels in an uproar," but scientists don't know the reason why.

One reliable observer swears that standing before a rack of books in a local library invariably results in the call to stool; another knows that merely the thought of a trip anywhere sends him straight to the bathroom. The most common event that stirs the rectum to a propulsive contraction is the everyday act of eating breakfast. For over a century physiologists have talked about the "gastrocolic reflex," that is, food entering the stomach also spurs the colon.

Although the gastrocolic reflex is thus a normal event that allows us to predict within minutes when our daily bowel movement will occur, nobody understands precisely how food in the stomach sets off the colon. Since the reflex is still observed in animals after all nerves from the stomach and colon have been severed, hormones as well as nerves must be involved. For many, the gastrocolic reflex is as predictable as the dawn and comes shortly after breakfast. For others the call will come when least expected.

Constipation

For most people with constipation, no disease exists and none will be found. Remember, your bowel moves with a *regular* rhythm and frequency of its own. The frequency of bowel movements may increase as you add more fiber to your diet, drink more water, or experience the stress of everyday life. Constipation, in contrast, is caused by the failure of the colon muscle to contract with the powerful thrust that makes up the urge to defecate. Think of constipation as more difficult or less frequent passage of stool than you are regularly accustomed to. To use laxatives because of constipation associated with a mild infection, a dietary fast, or mental depression does nothing to improve health, although millions of rational people believe exactly the opposite. "Be good and do your duty," many adults recall hearing as children. They strained and tried to comply. In this way did a simple biologic act become a lifelong preoccupation for a substantial number of otherwise healthy persons.

The second result of the "good-bad" form of toilet training is that any subsequent variation on regularity or promptness is perceived as abnormal. As with other natural acts that are better simply done than ruminated about, dwelling upon having a "normal" bowel movement makes this goal as unattainable for millions as does running the four-minute mile. Much as the insomniac who moans, "I can't go to sleep; I will never be able to go to sleep!" and thus ensures sleeplessness, a minor change in bowel habit toward constipation often arouses concern that seems to suppress the colon more than before.

When constipation occurs, the body in general often

becomes the focus of extraordinary—even unwarranted—attention, and many people sense fatigue, experience headaches, and worry increasingly not *whether* slowed bowel function is related to their symptoms, but *how.* Such concerns propel people who are worried about their health into physicians' waiting rooms everywhere. Doctors hear these complaints so frequently, and so rarely discover a true illness, that many simply respond that there is "no organic disease" present and acquiesce to the patients' desire for regularity. The laxative manufacturers are pleased to oblige. Each advertisement links yesterday's clouds to constipation or the euphemistic "irregularity," and today's sunny disposition therefore results from the use of the recommended product that cleared both the colon and the emotional weather. It's a persuasive marketing strategy even though medical support for the logic employed simply doesn't exist.

This pervasive idea linking regularity to health is related to another that takes on some of the aspects of a social taboo. Even in modern society, where such formerly "hidden" topics as sex and divorce are now openly discussed, the mere mention of the bowels results in awkward responses. It's something we're expected to worry about but not speak of. Comedians make us laugh at the subject but the endless jokes about defecation, feces, gas, and hemorrhoids put us on our guard when we enter a doctor's office. Even when the most tactful, sympathetic doctor asks what the trouble is, some patients fear that their complaints will be dismissed with a jest. Keep in mind that it's not a laughing matter to doctors, nor is it a mark of primitive behavior to worry aloud about the bowels.

Some causes of persistent constipation can be uncovered by a doctor who considers problems like low thyroid function, psychiatric depression, dehydration, narcotic overuse, or a tumor that obstructs the colon itself. Temporary constipation may result simply from the unavailability of a familiar toilet; travel can thus induce either diarrhea as *turista,* or constipation of startling intensity and duration. If you have sought relief of constipation by seeing a physician, a good doctor will take a careful history and perform a complete physical examination, including a thorough rectal examination. If a doctor merely prescribes laxatives without this rectal exam, he is not doing his job properly. Of course, you may feel that you are not "doing your job properly" and that the few days without a bowel movement signify serious disease. That is simply not the case. By drinking six full glasses of water a day, adding more fiber to the diet, and setting aside a few more minutes each morning for quiet and contemplation, even stubborn constipation may yield. In these matters, the change in bowel *habit* is more important than frequency. If you've had a "one stool every other day" bowel habit for ten years and then suddenly experience either continued diarrhea or constipation, see your doctor.

When we are healthy, our bowel habit—the digestive events in the small bowel and the drying and emptying events in the colon—is dependable. But, just as we take the normal functioning of our hearts for granted until someone hears a heart murmur or we develop chest pain, so the dull colon becomes a focus for intense concentration should we develop colon cancer or a thrombosed hemorrhoid or ulcerative colitis. With pain and a change in bowel habit, we suddenly become very much aware of what we've taken for granted up till that time. Several medical problems of the bowel are discussed in subsequent chapters of this book, both minor annoyances like *turista* and hemorrhoids, and serious diseases like diverticulitis and cancer, as well as the apparent problems that make life so miserable for perfectly normal people—gas or a fluctuating bowel habit. Yet remember that for all the concern we may have with the colon and its product, the life-giving process of digestion does not require the presence of the colon at all.

3
Apparent Colon Disease

Apparent colon disease is a term that refers to an enigma in the practice of medicine wherein a person experiences symptoms that seem to point to a diagnosis of disease in the colon, yet a competent physician, careful and thorough in evaluating the patient, finds none. The common symptoms of such patients include constipation, diarrhea, or alternating episodes of each, often accompanied by mild to moderate abdominal pain. These symptoms often recur in episodic form over a period of many months or years. The physician will search *in vain* for evidence of colon disease by asking about rectal bleeding, fever, severe pain with nausea or vomiting, and by examining the patient for masses in the belly, ulcers in the wall of the rectum or colon, malnutrition, or anemia. Further examination involves either inserting into the rectum tubes with illuminated tips that explore the rectum, sigmoid area, and the entire colon (thus called sigmoidoscopes or colonoscopes), or giving barium as an enema.

Gastroenterologists are experts in colon disease, and they report being confronted daily with the enigma of apparent colon disease in patients who consult them after other physicians have referred them to "an expert." Many patients feel relieved that cancer or ulcerative colitis is not present, and learn to live with their symptoms. Others seek the advice of surgeons, undergo exploratory operations, and a few months later experience a return of the initial symptoms and begin another expensive and frustrating cycle of seeking an answer.

This perplexing riddle of symptoms without disease can be examined from a somewhat different perspective. As the previous chapter described, most people possess in the gastrointestinal tract a superbly efficient organ system. The first thirty-five feet or so, from the mouth through the stomach into the small bowel and to the beginning of the colon, are concerned solely with the process of digesting food, water, and salts. One could subsist for a year on a vitamin-supplemented diet of peanut butter, carrots, and milk; or one of fish, rice, and sweetened tea; or any of thousands more; and manage to keep each of the trillions of cells in the human body normal and healthy. The small bowel digests what it can—which is nearly everything that enters—and the liquid indigestible leftovers enter the colon to be dried and thickened during a leisurely trip that ends with a splash and a sigh.

The major business of the whole bowel, digestion, is finished before the colon ever commences its act; so the removal of solid waste via defecation can occur *normally* twice a day or once a week in equally healthy people. Considering the variation in frequency of this biologic event, one man's constipation may be another's diarrhea. Diarrhea is usually defined as a condition in which unformed stools are passed more frequently *than normal,* and constipation is difficult passage of stool less often *than normal.* Normal for you and me, that is, and not for each and every member of the family of man.

Recall that we leave the small bowel out of this discussion altogether, and talk now only about the drying tank of the colon. Millions have an *apparent* colon disease (ACD) because of one or more symptoms—say constipation—without a shred of objective evidence to confirm the diagnosis of true disease. The key word is "apparent."

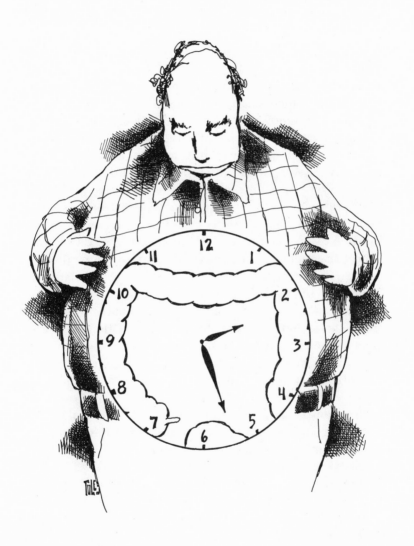

Your colon may be fine and work fine, but it doesn't "seem" to. What "seems" but isn't is "functional" to physicians. With functional disorders, cells are normal. For example, headaches may cause disabling pain, even suggesting a brain tumor, but a brain tumor is not found. No one doubts that headaches truly hurt, but most are due simply to tension, not tumor. In medicine the term "organic" describes disease that "is," and can be verified under the pathologist's microscope.

Some examples of possibly functional problems include backache, headache, obesity, some itchy rashes, hypoglycemia, irregular or painful menses, lassitude, and fatigue. All are common symptoms or conditions and cause their sufferers to restrict their lifestyle, miss work, and seek professional help for diagnosis and treatment. Each of these problems may represent the first symptom of serious organic disease, but usually an organic disease isn't found. The patients then find relief by a variety of methods— some quite peculiar—and others rejoice that their health is good and simply go on living. It's impressive how often the latter attitude brings the relief so fervently and unsuccessfully sought by more troublesome tactics, including visits to one doctor after another.

When colon symptoms occur, there is genuine concern that real disease has begun, whether cancer or ulcerative colitis. Yet, for most people with colon symptoms (who seem to have something wrong with the colon), no blood is seen in the stool, there is no weight loss, the appetite is good, and overall health is unimpaired. The enigma exists because symptoms of colon disease persist even though the rectum feels smooth to the doctor's exploring finger, and through a sigmoidoscope or colonoscope the internal wall of the rectum and colon—the mucosa—is seen to be pink, healthy, and normal, free of cancer, ulcer, or bleeding. If a barium enema is carried out to complete the evaluation, the x-rays too are "negative." "Negative" in this regard refers to health and "positive" to disease.

Since some symptoms referable to the colon—say pain—can in fact be caused by diseases involving the pancreas, kidneys, spine, or uterus, a conscientious physician considers and tests for disease in areas elsewhere. After such a negative evaluation, then, you may be reassured that your colon complaint—whether cramps or constipation—is not due to organic disease. Yes, the symptom may be troubling and certainly inconvenient, but the doctor is reassuring for good reason—no disease is present that may shorten your life. The dilemma, of course, is that good news—no disease—leads to a question in so many people, "Fine, but then what *is* the trouble?"

Some Colon Stories
That Perplex Doctors and Patients

We will sound a few common themes of normal and healthy people who suffer the enigma of symptoms without disease. Their bowel symptoms are troubling enough to bring them back to physicians again and again as they seek a diagnosis, or at least relief. First is a young man of thirty-five, with diarrhea on shopping day, or when he overbooks reservations in his small French restaurant. Should the dishwasher grumble about work and talk of leaving, the owner's bowels roar and send him racing to the bathroom. Later, perhaps, a similar restaurant opens up nearby, or the economic recession deepens, so that empty tables appear more frequently. The bowel habit abruptly switches to one of bitter constipation. The restaurant owner might even accept diarrhea again if only his customers would return. There is nothing crazy about him at all—save that his colon became the target organ for the expression of stress he feels. Others might experience headaches, muscle aches, fatigue, or painful and irregular menstrual periods. Many more drink, swallow drugs, work harder, or brood about precisely what's wrong and why they feel this way.

Next consider a woman, "regular" by virtue of laxatives, enemas, and bran, who started her own daughter on soapsuds enemas at the age of three or four, and years later accompanies her into the doctor's office. The mother sounds the complaint of constipation in her now adolescent daughter. The daughter is ashamed, silent, and appears depressed. What is wrong?

The next patient is a venture capitalist, a type A personality from his squeaking shoes to the graying tips of his tightly curled hair. A man separated from his wife and now living with a much younger woman, he seems very "laid back" in demeanor—and yet with "this new phase of my existence," as he terms it, he has returned to the bowel habits he recalls as a very young boy. Hectic diarrhea now occurs before every important conference, as before kindergarten class years ago, and meetings are sometimes postponed as our entrepreneur frantically occupies himself in wiping and wiping again.

On a Monday morning while shaving, he has the urge to move his bowels even before breakfast but passes little save a small amount of watery stool. He leaves his penthouse apartment having moved his bowels four to six times, and his sore bottom makes him a slightly less jaunty figure than his business associates have come to expect. From Monday noon until Thursday his colon is entirely silent. He scheduled the appointment with the gastroenterologist for the next Monday, and even after three smallish, watery movements, his rectum still contained feces instead of being empty after defecation, as it should be. In contrast to the previously described restaurateur, who recognizes that his colon is his target organ, this sophisticated man rejects all such suggestions. These "so-called doctors" have a lot more to learn, he states.

Several forms of apparent colon disease cause symptoms of pain or aching more than those of diarrhea or constipation. In one of these, symptoms arise from stool and gas momentarily bunched together in the colon at the left upper part, near the location of the spleen. The pain spreads from the colon, where it began, up into the left rib cage and sometimes suggests a heart attack.

Some other examples of colon pain seem minor by contrast, but not if the symptoms lead to unnecessary surgery. In women whose abdominal muscles are lax from the physical strain of several pregnancies, who are unused to exercise and are taking laxatives, vague pains may spread from the colon to other parts of the abdomen, and the surgical removal of normal gall bladders and pelvic organs may result. Adhesions sometimes develop after surgery, by the way, and these thin strands of scar tissue can cause nagging pains or heaviness in the abdomen. Laxatives lead to bowel movements and the pain disappears. Can there be any doubt that such patients will continue the laxative habit for many years? More important, how will the busy doctor's statement, "Your colon is perfectly normal; just cut out the laxatives," sound to such a person? A surgeon who suggests additional surgery "to break up the adhesions" may find his suggestion eagerly accepted by patients tired of pain and perfunctory reassurance.

Here are some additional brief sketches of complaints by troubled people with altered bowel habits. *Each of them has a colon free of disease.*

1. Irregular timing of defecation with cramps before and relief after.

2. Constipation on weekends; diarrhea Monday; a normal stool Wednesday.

3. The urgent feeling that without a toilet *now* pants will be soiled.

4. A variation of the urgency: rapid defecation is followed in a few minutes by the urge to go again.

5. The laxative used to be required only every week or so, but is now necessary every other day.

6. The act of proper defecation requires an elaborate ritual. It begins with the preparation of the bathroom— spreading newspapers about, certain music, the right time of day—and so on until the relaxation of the anus and the act itself can occur. The postlude is only slightly shorter, including, among other stages, the inspection of the product, the folding of paper and wiping and patting each quadrant, then the flush, and the surgical scrub of hands and forearms before windows are opened and air deodorizers cover all with an unnatural scent. The prelude alone can last up to thirty minutes, and a single knock on the bathroom door or the ringing of the phone cancels everything, and necessitates starting over.

7. Sweating and light-headedness before, during, or after the passage of an otherwise normal stool, often leaving the passer exhausted and near-fainting.

8. The irresistible urge to defecate before important appointments or any major personal event.

9. Alternating periods of diarrhea and constipation with normal health.

10. The passage of strands of mucus that resemble worms or fibers.

11. The devout conviction that today's fatigue and mental sluggishness result directly from retained stool. The only clear result of this widely held belief is a laxative market that exceeds $250 million a year in the United States alone.

12. Rectal pain that awakens young people, usually men aged eighteen to thirty-five, and slowly subsides. It returns at intervals in the succeeding week. A cause is not found.

13. A "nervous" stomach with fluttering pains around the navel present immediately upon waking. Since the sufferers use the word "stomach," a number of them swallow

barium, yet nothing abnormal is found when x-rays are examined.

14. *Any* of the above accompanied by brief, sharp, grunt-producing pain that lasts for a few seconds, changes in location, and totally disappears after defecation.

The Frequency and Cause of Apparent Colon Disease

Some professionals estimate that at least a quarter of all adults experience functional colon symptoms. Yet fewer than a third of these troubled people ever see a doctor. It seems a testimony to our basic common sense that temporary variations in bowel habits do not propel us to a doctor's office. Blood in the stool, severe pain, or fever require prompt diagnosis, however.

Those with functional complaints who do see a doctor (or doctors) may bring photographs of what has appeared in the toilet lately, or they arrive with thick notebooks that annotate the bowel habit in bizarre detail. Others do not voice their complaint as much as show it. Paper bags are unwrapped and out come fruit jars, milk cartons, plastic dry-cleaning bags and wide-mouth bottles, all surrounding or covering stools. People who doctor-shop sometimes become very hostile as they recall the time and money spent in search of an answer and the frustrating failure to find an effective one. Reassurance that "there's nothing really wrong" is so at variance with the sense of concern that the patient simply intensifies his or her determination to find the real truth. After all, some constipation indeed results from early cancer of the colon or rectum, and colitis—true ulcerative colitis—invariably begins with diarrhea. Further, we now have learned that most diarrhea of travelers is due to bacterial infection, not anxiety, and low thyroid function can cause constipation. So the "apparent" aspect of colon trouble, the doctor shoppers conclude, is due in large part to the incompetence of physicians or the primitive state of medical science. Thousands of them therefore consult yet another physician, or a chiropractor, or a homeopath—and try almost anything to achieve the distant goal of normality or regularity.

Consider the case of a young woman. A superbly organized nurse, she had apparently experienced lifelong variations in her bowel habit. While considering a marriage proposal from a man about whom she had mixed feelings, she developed abdominal cramps, diarrhea, and extreme weakness. Her doctor, a general practitioner, admitted her to a hospital to be observed for possible appendicitis. She didn't have appendicitis. A barium enema of the colon showed some spasm "but nothing organic," and no ulcers suggesting true ulcerative colitis were seen on sigmoidoscopic exam.

Melanie (a fictional name) returned to work, having been told that she had "mucous or spastic colitis," and she now took medicines that included sulfa drugs, a tranquilizer, and a stool softener. What Melanie did *not* receive was a strong, reassuring statement that her colon was intrinsically healthy and that she did not suffer from organic disease. What she needed most was a sympathetic approach to her functional problem, not a fistful of plastic medicine vials. I suggested the name of a gastroenterologist to her, if she wanted another opinion. She did not follow my suggestion.

I do not know what happened to Melanie, although she married and moved away. Very likely she remains convinced that she suffers from true colitis, and if her new doctor sees the sulfa pills and hears of her hospital admission, he may believe it as well. Thousands of sufferers want a precise reason for symptoms, and doctors who search for it use terms like spastic colitis, a touch of colitis, mucous colitis, intestinal malfunction, or abnormal adhesions causing colitis.

Why does the colon, in its everyday work, cause such disturbing symptoms in so many people? We know at least a few of the reasons. Some colon symptoms arise from a crucial action of this organ—muscle contraction. We know that the wall of the colon is a muscle and so contracts and relaxes as does every other muscle. The colon is also in motion most of the time as water is absorbed from the contents that are slowly traveling along, propelled by contractions.

Any muscle that contracts and relaxes does so with the discharge of electricity (hence the name *electrocardiograph* for the instrument which measures the activity of the heart muscle). Probes have been inserted to monitor this electrical activity in human colon muscle, and they reveal that some patients with "functional" diarrhea show increased numbers of three-cycle-per-minute electrical waves. But no precise link has been found to prove that increased electrical activity in the muscle wall increases the number of bowel movements. Part of the colon, like the midpart of a long snake, may be contracting even as segments above and below relax.

As muscles contract, by the way, a sensation of pain may occur—labor pains after all are due to the contracting muscular wall of the uterus. The heart muscle contracts seventy times a minute, and most of us feel nothing, but if you lie on your left side and worry about your heart, the painful thumping will keep you awake. As worry subsides, so do the anxiety and the rhythmic thumping. For those with painful contractions of the colon, the pain takes different forms, and varies in intensity from a flutter to a stab. Laxatives themselves can cause pain by increasing the intensity of muscular contractions of the colon, but they do organize muscle and electrical activity to get the colon's "act" together.

One of the true experts on apparent colon disease is Dr. T. P. Almy, who has studied the problem and viewed medical progress for over three decades. He has written:

"Disturbances of colon function characteristic of the irritable colon are normal bodily manifestations of emotional tension analogous to sweating, facial flushing, and weeping." Dr. Almy has inserted balloonlike devices through the rectums of willing volunteers as they rested, discussed unemotional matters, and later talked of intimate and personal problems. The electrical impulses and muscle responses of the colon wall *did* react to changes in the emotional states, but sadly no predictable pattern was found.

How to Live with Colon Symptoms

Here are ten suggestions that may be useful. The first is the most important.

1. If bloody or black stools or severe pain in the abdomen occurs, get competent help as soon as possible. In a strange city, head for the emergency room of the largest hospital in town. If constipation or diarrhea or pain, with or without loss of weight, began less than three months ago, see a good, thoughtful physician. Pick a specialist in internal or family medicine who is willing to spend at least forty-five minutes taking your medical history and examining you. The examination must include a rectal exam and a search for blood in the stool. Further testing may well involve a sigmoidoscopy, or x-rays with barium enema, or barium swallowed to view the upper gastrointestinal tract. Blood tests and a chest x-ray are best included in a complete evaluation.

One other point is worth remembering. If your colon symptoms have lasted for six months or longer and an evaluation of the kind described above is negative, the chance that your symptoms signify serious or progressive disease is virtually zero.

2. (This and the following eight suggestions assume that symptoms have been present for months or years and no disease has been diagnosed.) If a specific food causes

Pain and Apparent Colon Disease

Nearly one of every two people who consult a doctor with any gastrointestinal complaint turns out to have no organic disease, and English investigators use the term "irritable bowel syndrome" to describe the symptoms, often painful, in such otherwise healthy people. An excellent article in the medical journal *Lancet* in 1980 reported on a group of these patients evaluated in a London clinic. After organic disease was excluded by a large number of tests, the patients consented to have a colonoscope inserted well up into their colons with a balloon attached and inflated with air. The patients were asked to describe where pain occurred, and if the pain was the same as that they originally felt.

Forty-eight patients were so studied, and the investigators reported:

- Colon symptoms had lasted an average of 4 years.
- Two-thirds had seen at least one other specialist for the same problem before.
- To investigate or "treat" the pain, 11 of 48 patients had undergone one operation, 4 had two, 2 had three, and one had been operated on four times.
- Of the operations performed, 10 were exploratory without organs being removed, but 7 patients had their gall bladders removed, 6 had hysterectomies, 3 had appendectomies, and 2 had ulcer operations.
- From 25 ml to 250 ml of air in the balloon (2 tablespoons to a cupful) caused symptoms exactly or very similar to the original pain in over half the patients. Most of these pains were felt in the lower abdomen, especially on the left side.
- As the balloon was inflated inside the colon, some of the pain occurred in such places as the back, lower ribs, and groin.

Conclusions: With normal colons, sporadic pain from apparent colon disease (irritable bowel) can last for years, be felt in various places, and leads to unnecessary surgery.

diarrhea or pain, stop eating it. Otherwise, eat what you want. Millions of people have given up food or drink they genuinely enjoy because they were told by a well-meaning amateur or professional that the particular substance was "no good for you." You can decide for yourself. Moderation deserves mention, for example, if you can handle two alcoholic drinks without any problems, whereas six cause diarrhea and pain, not to mention headache and silly behavior.

3. Lactose, the sugar in milk and milk products, is the commonest food that causes diarrhea, pain, and gas, because of a true failure to digest it (see box on page 36). Since more than 25 percent of American adults have lactose intolerance, omit milk products if they cause symptoms. Cut out milk drinking first; you may not have to omit cheese, yogurt, or ice cream, but some people must be alert to the lactose present in many foods, and learn to avoid them.

4. If your complaint is primarily constipation, and not diarrhea, add more fiber to your diet. These plant-derived substances cannot be digested by animal guts like ours (see Fiber, page 52). As a result the undigested fiber will increase the weight of stool passed, soften it as more water stays in the colon, and will increase the frequency of defecation. If you don't care for bran cereal, try shredded wheat, which contains only about a quarter as much fiber as bran cereal but still exceeds the amount in the diet of most of us. Aside from breads, crackers, and cereals, you may try vegetables high in fiber, namely carrots, corn, parsnips, kidney beans, peas, and summer squash. Fruits rich in fiber include apples, blueberries, pears, and strawberries. A natural nonfood product is a preparation of psyllium seeds (Metamucil is one brand). Drink it with a whole glass of water three times a day. Whichever form of fiber you take, give it a reasonable trial, say a month, before discarding it. If cereal with milk causes burning diar-

rhea, you have diagnosed lactose intolerance in yourself. In that case, eat bran baked in muffins.

5. Drink enough water. Remember that the colon is very efficient in extracting water from the moving column of waste, and stony stools hurt. Most of us, as we age, drink less fluid than we should. One swallow of water from the drinking fountain does not equal a glassful, by the way. Some experts praise warm water; others, distilled or bottled. The type of water is less important than the quantity.

6. Allow time for the bowels to move and a little more time for them to move completely. Many constipated souls feel nothing until just as they race out of the house or get on a bus. Help your healthy colon work naturally. Drink a whole glassful of warm water and then eat breakfast. Allow at least 20 minutes in private, seated silence in the bathroom after breakfast, perhaps reading. Try this approach every day for at least two weeks before deciding that, like the others, these simple measures can't really work. If you would rather sleep the extra twenty minutes, you have a problem mild enough to ignore all this advice.

7. Keep your bowel complaints to yourself. Loved ones may claim differently, but they no longer want to hear. If some of these suggestions help you, do announce the good news to those who have borne your sorrows so uncomplainingly themselves. Their positive comments will only reinforce your new approach.

8. Stop using stimulant laxatives and enemas. Fiber is a natural laxative and can take the place of all the medicines that induce artificial "regularity" while actually unbalancing a very complex organ—the human gastrointestinal tract. If you must resort to an enema every now and then, use plain tap water—soap can cause inflammation of the colon lining.

9. If you are constipated and decide to break a laxa-

Milk and Intestinal Symptoms

Lactose is the main sugar (carbohydrate) in milk and milk products, and the sugar is digested after it is broken down by the enzyme lactase present in the lining cells of the small bowel. Probably 15% of white adults and 50% of black adults lack the lactase necessary to digest milk sugar. Several points about this common problem deserve emphasis:

1. The failure to digest lactose is caused by a hereditary or inborn lack of the enzyme lactase, yet for unknown reasons the symptoms don't develop until the age of puberty or later.

2. Bacteria in the small bowel and colon break down undigested lactose to hydrogen and other gases. The undigested sugar also draws water into the intestine. These two events give rise to the symptoms of lactose intolerance that include one or more of the following:
   a. Diarrhea   c. Cramps
   b. Gas   d. Bloating

3. A juice glass full of milk (100 cc. or 4 oz.) contains 5 grams of lactose, enough to cause symptoms. Skim milk has less fat but no less lactose than whole milk. Ice cream, cheeses, and yogurt contain varying amounts.

4. The diagnosis of lactose intolerance can be confirmed by showing that blood-sugar levels fail to rise after a dose of lactose is given by mouth. This sugar isn't being digested.

5. Since lactase deficiency may first cause symptoms in young adulthood, you may have milk intolerance now even if you drank gallons of milk without problems as a youngster.

6. Some adults labeled as having the "irritable bowel syndrome" or apparent colon disease will improve dramatically if milk is omitted from the diet. Some "nondairy" milk substitutes contain lactose, so check labels to avoid errors.

7. The inability to digest lactose is not the same as "milk allergy." That problem is seen in infants who are allergic to the *protein* in milk and so develop skin rashes, feeding problems, and diarrhea. Lactose intolerance is due to a failure to digest a sugar, not an allergy to a protein.

tive habit, you may not have a bowel movement for seven days or ten days or even twenty days. The material accumulating in your colon is *not* dangerous to your health. Anticipate and accept the twinges and the distended belly that will result. It is worth the wait.

10. You have likely heard from a doctor that you have irritable bowel syndrome, spastic colitis, mucous colitis, or a "functional" bowel problem. If the examination included a careful rectal exam, a sigmoidoscopy and an x-ray with a barium enema, and ulcerative colitis or cancer was not found, be assured that your colon is *normal*, no matter how unusual your symptoms or bowel habits seem to be.

4
Laxatives, Enemas, and Fiber

Laxatives, enemas, and fiber sound three variations on the single theme of regularity. For every person who takes a vitamin capsule once a day in the belief that this medicine maintains health, someone else starts breakfast with a bran cereal or swallows a laxative at bedtime or self-administers an enema. In fact, for those who take a vitamin and have a bowel movement each morning, the in-out cycle must seem an ideal way to maintain health. The regularity may be achieved by substances that many people refer to as cathartics or purgatives, terms that refer to cleansing and purification of something negative or harmful. Every drugstore carries fifty such products, many available without a prescription, and all are advertised in newspapers and on television as safe and effective. The desire for regularity and the "safe" ways to achieve it account for the continuing popularity of a whole group of drugs. Women use laxatives much more often than men do, and laxative use increases with age. With chronic use, more medicine is needed to "get the job done," and so recommended doses of laxatives are routinely exceeded. Those who take enemas regularly are invariably women who learned the ritual at a very early age and have maintained it ever since. Younger people who seek regularity in "natural" ways have added more fiber to the daily diet, and so continue the tradition started by the grandmother who ate bran cereal and whole-wheat bread for the "roughage" that kept her colon regular.

Each of these approaches used to stimulate the colon muscle or clear the colon will be discussed separately.

Laxatives

The contents of the colon move in but one direction, provided that it is not completely obstructed by cancer or twisted upon itself. Laxatives speed the flow by lubricating the contents, by wetting them, or by stimulating the muscle wall of the colon to contract more often and more vigorously. Nearly all laxatives are derived from the plant world. You may think that oil derived from the castor bean is a lubricant but castor oil works by irritating the muscular wall of the colon, and is so correctly classified as a true bowel stimulant. Another laxative formerly derived from the plant world is cascara sagrada, literally "sacred bark." The garden also yields up laxative substances from rhubarb as well as senna and aloe. Both cascara and senna are now usually derived from coal tar. Phenolphthalein derives from the may apple, its bitter taste masked by chocolate, and it is sold as Ex-Lax.

Many of these laxatives stimulate the colon muscle to contract, a harsh action by definition, and users often experience additional contractions, and the urge to defecate, even after the act has taken place. Thus a laxative-induced bowel movement may be followed by rumbling and cramps that last for hours, with the repeated passage of small stools. The cleaning-out process also causes the loss of a rather large amount of liquid in the stool, which must be made up by drinking more water. Since bowel movements induced by laxatives can weigh a kilogram or more (2 pounds) and since the world nowadays puts such a premium on a slim figure, young ladies preparing for the

Laxatives

Class	What they are
Bulk or bulk-forming	Complex sugars (polysaccharides) Plant-derived fibers (cellulose) or seed-derived (psyllium)
Stool softeners	Wetting and dispersing agents (usually the salt dioctyl sodium sulfosuccinate or dioctyl calcium sulfosuccinate)
	Mineral oil (indigestible oil from petroleum)
Stimulant or contact	1. Castor oil (from seeds of *Ricinus communis*)
	2. Bisacodyl (a diphenyl methane compound)
	3. Phenolphthalein (a diphenylmethane compound)
	4. Anthraquinones (senna, cascara sagrada, danthron)
Salts	Magnesium salt and phosphates or sulfates

What they do	Trade names	Safety notes/Possible problems (see text)
Dissolve or swell in water Draw water into colon	Metamucil, Serutan, Konsyl, Modane-Bulk, Syllact	Quite safe—take with a full glass of water
Lowers surface tension to allow water and fat to enter colon	Colace, Modane-Soft, Surfak	Quite safe; be alert for combinations: Peri-Colace (casanthranol *added*) Doxidan (danthron *added*) Correctol (phenolphthalein *added*)
Lubricant	Agoral Plain	Agoral Raspberry (phenolphthalein *added*)
Stimulates *small bowel* and colon	Neoloid	Best used under a physician's care
Stimulates colon when taken by mouth or in rectal suppository	Carter's Little Pills Dulcolax	May cause cramps, burning
Stimulates colon	Ex-Lax	Red stool or urine, skin rashes
Mechanism not precisely known	Senokot tablets; Modane tablets and liquid	Melanosis coli (see text)
Partly absorbed; that remaining draws water into bowel	Epsom salt (magnesium sulfate) Phillips Milk of Magnesia (magnesium hydroxide suspended in water)	Avoid if kidney disease— may cause magnesium toxicity.
	Glauber's salt (sodium sulfate)	Avoid if heart failure or on salt-restricted diet

prom or a modeling career and boxers trying to make the weight can become and remain avid laxative users.

Types of Laxatives

The table on pages 40–41 lists four classes of laxatives in terms of what they are, what they do, some examples of trade names of marketed products, and a comment about possible side effects.

The first two classes are relatively safe drugs, but keep in mind that the laxative habit is easy to begin, very difficult to break, and laxatives are not needed to maintain health.

1. Bulk or bulk-forming agents, being the safest form of laxatives, are listed first. These complex sugars are essentially indigestible fibers derived from plants. Rather than directly stimulating the colon muscle to contract, they simply pass undigested into the colon and once there attract water into it. The fibers add bulk and water, and it is this "mass" or bulk of material that ultimately travels to the rectum and leads to the muscle contraction that initiates the bowel movement. The subject of dietary fiber is discussed in detail later in this chapter.

2. A second class of laxatives is not composed of fibers but of wetting or dispersing agents that allow water and fat to enter the colon and soften the stool.

These two classes of laxatives are safe, mild, and can be used for long periods of time without side effects. However, both bulk laxatives and stool softeners draw water out of the rest of the body, so people taking any laxative in these classes should drink at least a glassful of water with the medicine, and four to six more glasses during the day. Alcoholic beverages do not provide the needed fluid because the alcohol acts on a body hormone and so allows for the excretion of more water as urine than is taken in as beer, wine, or liquor. This fact about alcohol explains the dehydration of the morning after, by the way.

A stool softener works safely but rather slowly and so a stimulant laxative is often combined with it. A seemingly minor change in drug name from Colace to Peri-Colace signifies a major change in product from a stool softener to a combination of stool softener *and* stimulant laxative. Mineral oil taken by mouth is simply a softening lubricant and so can help those who pass hard stool, an often painful process. Agoral Plain is mineral oil, but Agoral Raspberry contains both mineral oil and phenolphthalein, the stimulant laxative also sold separately as Ex-Lax. The table below shows some of these combinations, and the table (pages 40–41) remarks (Safety Notes) on the same thing.

The phrase *combination of ingredients* has the sound of a scientific product, one tailor made to fit a precise need, but drugs interact in sometimes startling and unforeseen ways. In general, the best medicine is the least medicine. This is even more pertinent in the case of laxatives, which are not necessary to cure disease or maintain health. Laxative combinations are therefore best avoided. Fortunately, few laxatives sold in the United States contain more than two separate chemical substances. In Europe and many Central American countries, however, the stimulant laxative *oxyphenisatin* is used alone or in combi-

Some Laxative Combinations

Brand Name	Constituents
Agoral Raspberry	Mineral oil; phenolphthalein (stimulant)
Correctol	Softener; phenolphthalein (stimulant)
Dialose Plus	Softener; casanthranol (stimulant)
Doxidan	Softener; anthraquinone (stimulant)
Haley's M-O	Magnesium salt; mineral oil (lubricant)
Peri-Colace	Softener; casanthranol (stimulant)
Senokot-S	Softener; senna (stimulant)

nation with several other drugs in multiple concoctions sold without a prescription. The drug oxyphenisatin causes chronic hepatitis and jaundice and its sale in the United States is now forbidden. When you are abroad, if the vendor of *any* laxative cannot prove by labeling that the proffered medicine is free of oxyphenisatin, don't buy it. The same advice holds for any proprietary drug sold over the counter anywhere to relieve gastrointestinal complaints. Consumers have every right to see a printed label that lists all ingredients present.

3. The most familiar laxative compounds are the stimulant or contact agents, listed on pages 40–41 as four different types, from castor oil to cascara. These laxatives directly stimulate the colon, and sometimes the small bowel as well. To "stimulate" means to make the muscle contract. The precise way in which this happens is not known, but Carter's Little Pills, Dulcolax, Ex-Lax, and Senokot tablets cause muscle contraction and the resulting propulsion of stool toward the rectum. Manufacturers may argue that one or the other stimulant may cause slightly less muscle contraction and so can be promoted as "gentle." Nevertheless, one gets the distinct feeling that the vendors are merely trying to sell their products. Castor oil, sold as the product Neoloid, stimulates the small bowel as well as the colon and is best used only under a doctor's care to prepare the bowel for examinations such as sigmoidoscopy or for barium enema. Possible side effects of stimulant laxatives include cramps with bisacodyl, skin rashes and red stool or urine with Ex-Lax, and a condition that results in a black colon wall, to be described. Laxatives are medicines, but users who routinely take twice or three times the recommended dose seem to ignore that fact.

4. The fourth type of laxative is one containing magnesium salts and phosphates or sulfates, and these salts draw water into the bowel. Epsom salt contains magnesium sulfate, whereas Phillips Milk of Magnesia is a suspension of magnesium hydroxide in water.

Sales figures of laxatives are jealously guarded trade

secrets, so it is impossible to know precisely which laxatives are the most used. However, as the total market for laxative products in the United States exceeds $250 million per year, not including fiber-rich cereals and breads, it is clear that many people regard these medicines as absolutely crucial for their well-being.

Are Laxatives Necessary?

No. The use of laxative combinations is problematic because two agents can cause more trouble than one. What about single-agent laxatives? Except for the rare situation where stool becomes compressed into a stone-hard mass that actually stops the colon, unpassed stool poses no risk to health whatsoever. Even if narcotic drugs have caused persistent constipation, stimulant laxatives and salts should not be used unless a fair trial with a bulking or softening agent fails.

Side Effects of Laxatives

1. If fever, abdominal pain or cramps, nausea, or vomiting is present, do not take any laxative for "relief." A disorder like appendicitis, true ulcerative colitis, or diverticulitis may be causing pain or nausea. In each of these situations, a laxative will cause contractions of an already inflamed and diseased part of the bowel. Using a laxative may thus result in perforation of the colon, a real disaster requiring emergency surgery to bring under control.

2. Older people and those with heart, liver, or kidney disease live in a complex balance with their body water, which contains several salts, including sodium, potassium, and magnesium. Any kind of laxative may alter this balance, sometimes abruptly.

Every physician can recall a patient whose heart disease worsened when sodium-containing laxatives (salts) were taken, or in whom laxatives caused diarrhea that depleted the body of potassium needed to maintain the normal rhythm of the heart. These preventable incidents occur far too often and demonstrate the subtle but serious problems that laxatives can cause, especially in older people.

3. The most startling complication of chronic laxative use is a condition known as melanosis coli, which means that a blackish pigment is found in the colon wall. Instead of being its normal healthy pink, the mucosa of the colon varies from medium brown to black. A biopsy will show that the cells of the mucous lining of the colon have become stuffed with a brownish-black pigment of unknown composition. Two anthracene laxatives, cascara and senna, which are derived from coal tar or plant substances, have been reported to color the colon in some carefully documented cases of melanosis coli. Further, an association between melanosis coli and cancer of the colon has been reported more than once. There is no scientific proof at this time that links one brand of laxative with discoloration of the colon wall. However, most experts recommend that any patient with a brownish-black appearance of the mucous membrane of the colon undergo a barium enema to help rule out colon cancer.

4. Women who have taken laxatives regularly for ten years or more may develop a condition called "cathartic colon." Owing to chronic use of the stimulant group of laxatives, the colon shortens and loses the normal scalloped curves of its wall. The result is impaired absorption of water and salt through the wall and ineffective muscle contractions. The afflicted women describe constipation, bloating, and vague pain in the lower abdomen. The abdomen is often distended as though the patient were swallowing air. On x-ray examination or colonoscopy, the colon appears waterlogged, and on barium enema examination, the appearance is that of organic ulcerative colitis, yet ulcers are not present.

Most physicians who diagnose melanosis coli or cathartic colon attempt to persuade their patients to stop laxative use altogether. In a surprising number of cases, the history of laxative abuse is denied, and the perplexed physician then urges a consultation with a gastroenterologist. Even when the specialist probes for the crucial information, chronic users of laxatives continue to deny the fact. The story of cathartic abuse remains a secret even when a biopsy specimen or barium examination proves otherwise. Consider the elements present: a compulsion to take cathartics; the dependence upon taking them; the need to increase the dose over a period of time to get the same effect; the withdrawal symptoms when they are no longer used; the denial of symptoms. All these are aspects of drug addiction, which explains why successful management of a patient with the problem of laxative abuse is so very difficult. In decades past, some patients with cathartic colon actually consented to a partial removal of the colon, even though removal of any part of the colon constitutes major surgery. Yet relief of constipation did not always follow. The cause of cathartic colon is not clear but some nerve cells in the colon wall are lost and so the motor activity—the true business of the colon—is interrupted.

The hopeful news for those afflicted by melanosis coli or cathartic colon is that changes *are* reversible if the use of cathartics and laxatives is stopped. If bulking or "natural" laxatives such as fiber are used instead, melanosis coli or cathartic colon won't develop or, if present, may improve. Bulk or bulk-forming laxatives or stool softeners are always preferable to laxatives of the stimulant, contact, or salt varieties.

No one has to take laxatives. Yet the habitual taking of laxatives at night is a personal ritual for millions of people. The notion persists that today's lassitude and fatigue will give way to tomorrow's brightened outlook if a laxative substance is used to clear the colon. The constant advertisements for "the gentle yet effective way to regularity" so favored by manufacturers of laxative products obviously reinforce this widely held belief.

To break the laxative habit requires the same courage needed to stop taking tranquilizers, sleeping pills, or even alcohol or cigarettes. And determination is even more important after laxative use stops. For the first several days of abstinence, bloating and a heavy dragging sensation may be prominent. In a person with lax abdominal muscles, the even more swollen appearance of the abdomen may seem too much to bear. So the medicine cabinet is reopened, and another cycle of laxative use begins.

You can shorten the waiting time for a drug-free bowel habit to redevelop by drinking six full glasses of water a day, and eating fiber in bran muffins and whole-wheat bread. Yet, even with enough water and plenty of fiber in the diet, the person who gives up the laxative habit may have to wait up to ten days before the truly natural action of the colon is re-established. It is worth restating that the retained colon product poses no risks, and breaking the habit is definitely worth the wait.

Enemas

Many people who never swallow laxatives (and some who do) will routinely "take" an enema, which is simply the injection of fluid into the rectum. The fluids used are plain water, soapy water, or water and salts sold in pre-packaged containers. As the fluid is held in the rectum for two or three minutes, increasingly vigorous contractions occur in the muscle of the lower colon, with the prompt evacuation of both fluid and stool.

An enema accomplishes from below within minutes what swallowed laxatives require eight hours to complete. Those who take enemas instead of laxatives do so out of habit, because "mother did it that way and she was always in good health," or because the cultural tradition of a cleansing ritual is an abiding one.

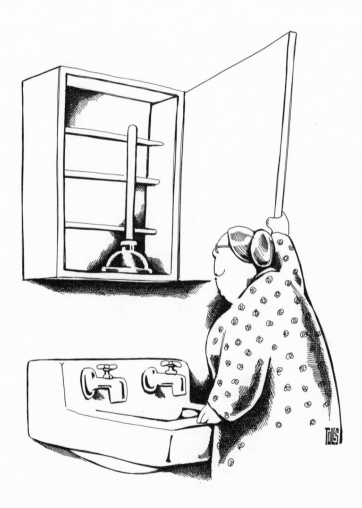

The most popular enema sold in America is the Fleet brand, a squeezable plastic container holding about four and a half ounces of sodium biphosphate and sodium phosphate and water. This salty water is inserted from the plastic container through a lubricated tip to increase bulk volume and water content of stool. The manufacturer states on the label that the product "usually produces evacuation within two to five minutes. Effectively relieves constipation and cleanses lower bowel." This statement about effectiveness, allowed by the Food and Drug Administration, has been interpreted by users as endorsement for the use of enemas. Words like *relieves* and *cleanses* recall others like *catharsis* and *purgation* so dear to laxative users, suggesting that regularity and well-being have a cause and effect relationship. The fact of the matter is that enemas *are* inexpensive and safe—unless appendicitis or diverticulitis is present—but should not be relied upon to maintain a regular bowel habit.

An enema is an important medical procedure when it is used to cleanse the bowel completely in preparation for the study of the colon with barium or a sigmoidoscope. If you are being evaluated for the cause of rectal bleeding, for example, castor oil is often prescribed the night before studies are scheduled. Unfortunately this stimulant laxative acts on both the small and large bowel and may result in explosive diarrhea three or four hours later, usually the middle of the night! To clean the colon entirely, another stimulant or contact laxative such as bisacodyl (Dulcolax) is given by mouth or inserted into the rectum to clean out what you thought the castor oil had already more than taken care of. The doctor may write an order for "plain water enemas until clear," these words meaning that you will receive enemas even after the castor oil and Dulcolax have worked. The intent is to rinse the colon of all fecal material. Several ounces of plain water repeatedly instilled into the rectum will cause the colon muscle to contract until no fecal matter is left and the fluid comes out as clear as it went in. A clean colon is crucial to allow for complete and unequivocal testing for disease. Every doctor has experienced the problem of a patient whose inadequately prepared colon retains lumps of feces that may resemble cancer when barium is introduced or obstructs the lighted instrument inserted to study the wall of the bowel for ulcers or cancer.

As stated before, enemas that contain plain water or water and phosphate salts are not dangerous to use unless a condition such as appendicitis or diverticulitis exists. In these situations, the already inflamed muscle contracts violently against the load of enema fluid presented, with severe pain or actual perforation of the colon a possible result. Doctors know of this danger, but quite a few are unaware that the use of soap in enemas to stimulate the colon further may possibly result in serious side effects. Even nowadays soap-suds enemas are ordered in many hospitals to prepare the patients for surgery or x-rays. However, soap is an irritant that will occasionally damage the lining cells of the colon to such an extent that severe abdominal pain and rectal bleeding occur. Worry about this dangerous form of colitis, known as soap colitis, has led many hospitals to abandon the use of soap-suds enemas and to substitute plain-water enemas, slightly less effective but much safer.

The printed warning on the Fleet brand enema states that "frequent or prolonged use of enemas may result in dependence." As with laxatives, the lifelong enema user simply can't give up his or, as is usually the case, her habits. For occasional use, a tap-water or packaged enema is safe, but remember that an enema interrupts the natural action of the colon itself as the salt and fluid unnaturally prod the colon to contract and result in a bowel movement. The daily ritual of the enema derives from the notion that retained stool is somehow unhealthful. It is not.

Until twenty years ago, some physicians used "high colonic irrigations" or enemas to empty virtually the entire colon in persons complaining of constipation, excess gas, and even backache and fatigue. The techniques employed were quite varied and sometimes bizarre, but the use of these "super-enemas" remained in vogue until physicians learned that the procedure has no medical value. Even as medical doctors (physicians) in America largely stopped prescribing this form of "treatment" in the last decade or so, several health spas in Europe have continued to offer high colonic enemas. A series of enemas to wash out the colon has also become popular among chiropractors and some nutritional counselors in the United States. A new and life-threatening danger of colonic irrigation has been described in the last few months. As reported from the Center for Disease Control (March 13, 1981), in a chiropractic clinic in Colorado no fewer than thirteen patients who underwent colonic irrigation developed infection with the agent that causes amebic colitis. Seven patients died, and health inspectors discovered that a contaminated machine had been used for the irrigations. This is a previously unrecognized complication of the "high colonic," a procedure that most health experts consider a medical fad to start with.

Fiber

Fiber, the indigestible latticework that keeps plants erect and apples and celery crisp, presently competes with jogging as one of the most popular drugless techniques to improve the health and well-being of today's adults. Breads are now stuffed with cellulose or shredded wood fiber, and television portrays the loving wife who chases after her man with the newest box of bran cereal in her grip. He is to eat it not because fiber is nutritious or inherently health-promoting, but because he may benefit from a laxative of the bulk or bulk-forming class. The purveyors of these laxatives, with one eye on the regulatory agencies

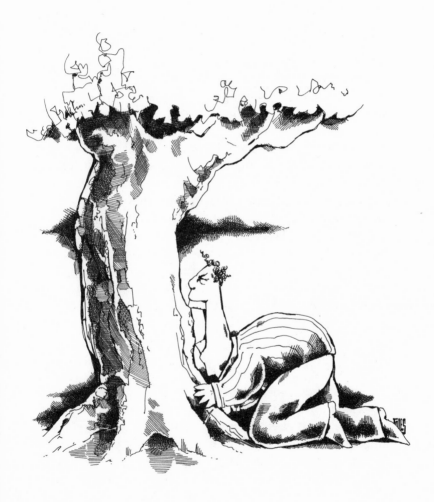

and the other on the expanded market for their products, first point out a truly natural way to promote a normal bowel habit, as cool mineral water is raised up out of a well in some verdant valley and drunk from an iron ladle. Lacking well water, we are urged to purchase fiber-rich substances such as All Bran, shredded wheat, or whole-wheat bread.

The crucial fact to remember about fiber, whatever its source, is that it qualifies as a laxative precisely because man's small bowel *cannot* digest it. No matter whether the fiber swallowed is cellulose in bran, fruit, and carrots; a woody substance called lignin, found in pears and potatoes; or gums from beans and oatmeal—our small bowel rejects them all and consigns them to the stream that flows into the colon. Bran cereal and many other high-fiber products are hailed as being rich in "dietary fiber," as though there were something wonderfully nourishing in the fiber present. There isn't. Dietary fiber is no more nutritious than is the cotton fiber sewn into shirts and blouses, or for that matter the cardboard that packages the brand of cereal you're now dutifully eating each morning.

But that's just the point. On entering the colon, undigested fiber is attacked by billions of bacteria that convert it to gas, water, and fats. Fats can't be digested in the colon and so simply lubricate what's present. The water prevents the stool from drying too much as it moves across and down the colon. The gas, mostly carbon dioxide, causes bloating and flatulence, but these two troubling side effects of a high-fiber diet subside within a few days. Cellulose fibers are not soluble in water at all, yet absorb a great deal of it, and so the stools of fiber eaters become much heavier and wetter. In this way more fiber in the diet leads to a bulky, moist, and easily passed stool without the aid of salts, stool softeners, or stimulant laxatives. This is about the view our great grandparents had, as they ate unpolished rice, whole-wheat bread, and plenty of raw fruits and vegetables. These foods and others listed in the accompanying box (page 55) kept people "regular" a cen-

Pros and Cons on the Value of More Fiber in the Diet

Pro	Con
1. Fiber adds bulk and water to stool without side effects.	1. Bacteria in the colon break down fiber to gas, with bloating and flatulence at least a temporary problem.
2. With less straining at stool, and better emptying, fiber helps those with hemorrhoids and constipation.	2. Agreed.
3. Bulky undigested fiber helps obese people lose weight.	3. For the elderly, or poorly nourished, the emphasis should be on a nutritious diet.
4. Dietary fiber is a safe and tasty food supplement.	4. "Dietary" fiber, since it goes undigested, is not a nutrient at all.
5. Fiber reduces the risk of diverticula becoming inflamed as diverticulitis.	5. A possible but unproven hypothesis.
6. Fiber will reduce the number of cases of colon cancer since cancer-causing substances will pass through the GI tract without being absorbed.	6. An outright speculation.
7. Since African villagers eating a high-fiber diet rarely suffer from heart disease and gallstones, the same may hold true for Western populations if eating habits are substantially altered.	7. Cause and effect relationships are difficult to prove and even then may not hold for other populations. In the meantime, food faddists who make major changes in the diet may experience new and unforeseeable health problems.

tury ago and are considered bulk or bulk-forming laxatives today.

The attitude of the medical community toward more dietary fiber is at present quite positive, as it was early in this century. The irony is that for twenty years after World War II medical opinion was just the reverse. At that time the trend in Western diets was to consume refined foods, such as white bread and polished rice, cooked fruits and vegetables (cooking reduces fiber content of some of these foods by half), and doctors took to recommending "low-roughage" diets for patients with a variety of conditions. It seemed logical that "roughage" would further aggravate the symptoms associated with an ulcer or diverticulitis. These refined diets low in fiber resulted in smaller stools passed with some difficulty. If constipation became a problem, the makers of laxatives were more than willing to provide relief with a growing variety of products. And the rich flocked to "health" spas whose principal attraction seemed to be high colonic enemas and purgatives taken in pleasant climates amid elegant company.

The logic of low-roughage "refined" diets unraveled as scientists learned that fibers don't further irritate any lining in the human gastrointestinal tract. In fact, undigested fiber speeds up almost all forms of movement in the small bowel and colon, adding water, bulk, and fat, the last split off from fiber by the action of bacteria in the colon. With this new information, the same physicians who advocated low-roughage diets twenty years ago now sagely suggest that more dietary fiber is a very good idea.

Two distinguished British physicians who also served in Africa, Drs. Hubert Trowell and Denis Burkitt, have been studying the effect of fiber for years and enthusiastically advocate its use. Dr. Trowell and his colleagues, by the way, coined the term "dietary fiber" in the medical journal *Lancet* in 1976, using the term to refer to any plant-derived complex sugar and woody fiber that passes through the GI tract of man undigested.

Drs. Burkitt and Trowell observed that Africans who regularly ate a diet high in dietary fiber were spared several medical disorders. Two of these diseases are bowel cancer and arteriosclerosis, the latter linked to excess fat in the blood. Many other scientists who have studied this area of digestion have confirmed that fiber certainly increases the bulk of the stool.

Since fiber eaters have more stool in the colon, the diameter of the organ must widen to accommodate its bulkier contents. At least one disease of the colon—diverticulitis—seems related to high pressure in its wall, and the greater the diameter of a tube such as the colon, the lower the pressure exerted. Africans rarely suffer from diverticulitis, and the British doctors seek more support for their idea that a diet high in fiber will reduce the colon pressure and so the risk. Since diverticula are present in the colons of nearly half the older population of America, and some of these outpouchings become inflamed to cause diverticulitis, a high-fiber diet may prevent formation of diverticula, or their inflammation.

Fiber also brings relief to hemorrhoid sufferers, who gratefully notice the resultant ease of defecation. Further, the complications of inflamed or thrombosed hemorrhoids may not occur. For those millions of people with apparent colon disease characterized by constipation, a greater weight of wet stool passing down the colon somewhat more rapidly seems an ideal form of therapy.

More extravagant claims about the value of fiber are being made, but these claims require hard data to support them. For example, take the supposition that if we eat cancer-producing chemicals in food, then the mild degree of failure of digestion (malabsorption) that occurs as undigested fiber speeds everything along may prevent the digestion of these cancer-causing substances. Trowell suggests that this explains the rarity of colon cancer in Africans, but others remain skeptical.

Can Fiber Cure Diabetes?

Dr. H. Trowell is one of two English physicians whose research and speculations helped fuel the explosive interest in dietary fiber. A few years ago he suggested that the absence of diabetes mellitus (the common kind) in African villagers correlated with their diet, one high in fiber. In the last two years, several articles in the medical literature have reported additional and rather startling information on this subject. In one small series of diabetic patients who required insulin for control of blood sugar, the need for insulin disappeared in most of them after they began eating a high-fiber diet. And the English journal *Lancet* published a report early in 1981 with the abridged title "A High . . . Fiber Diet Improves All Aspects of Diabetic Control." A more recent editorial in the same journal suggests caution "until this matter can be settled" (February 21, 1981, page 424).

Without taking either side of this rapidly growing controversy, a few facts are worth stressing:

- Dietary fiber is not absorbed, and so increases the weight and bulk of stool. Most people who stick with a high-fiber diet lose weight because the indigestible dietary fiber fills the stomach and leads to a feeling of satiety. Fiber may also slow the digestion of other foodstuffs, including fat. Perhaps half of all diabetics are overweight when the disease first appears. Every diabetes expert therefore counsels patients that weight loss down to "ideal" weight is the first step in the control of diabetes. The natural conclu-

Or consider that the digestion of fats such as cholesterol and triglycerides may contribute to arteriosclerosis and gallstones. The proof that a high-fiber diet impairs fat absorption *and therefore* spares man from disorders like these is probably years away, but the theoretical arguments sound convincing. The zeal of fiber proponents is exemplified by some recent comments about fiber and dision is that more fiber in the diet helps promote weight loss, and the now thin patient can be managed with less insulin, or none at all.

- The high-fiber diet that improved "all aspects of diabetic control" involved much more than merely adding a bran muffin or two to a normal diet. Breakfast for these patients included 5 ounces of beans a day, and the supper required nearly as much. Half a pound of beans a day represents a major change in eating habits for most people. Some would call it food faddism.

- Diabetes is a lifelong disease, yet the scientific studies that most enthusiastically support the value of fiber describe patients followed for fifteen months or less. Experts in this disease recall that many years ago the preferred diet for diabetics was one high in fat and low in carbohydrates. Two decades later, the preferred diet was precisely the opposite. The experts therefore want much more information before either climbing aboard the fiber bandwagon or overturning it.

- Unsupervised dieting is risky for diabetics taking insulin or other sugar-lowering drugs, because insulin reactions (hypoglycemia) may occur as food intake falls. Obese diabetics should therefore first consult the physician, and then lose excess weight by eating less of the foods they normally eat. Only then should a diet high in fiber be tried.

abetes, summarized in the box above. Doctors who know how rapidly fashions in medical practice can develop and fade remain understandably cautious as the fiber story is repeated with growing enthusiasm.

One clear benefit of eating indigestible fiber that draws water into the GI tract is the sensation of fullness achieved with less caloric intake. More fiber can thus be

Total Dietary Fiber in Selected Foods*

Food	Portion Size	Total Dietary Fiber/Serving (grams)
Breakfast Cereals		
All Bran	¾ cup	11.2
Cornflakes	¾ cup	2.1
Grapenuts	¾ cup	1.9
Rice Krispies	¾ cup	0.9
Special K	¾ cup	0.6
Bread		
Whole-wheat	1 slice	2.0
Brown	1 slice	1.2
White	1 slice	0.6
Vegetables (leafy)		
Broccoli tops (boiled)	½ cup	3.0
Brussels sprouts	½ cup	2.0
Cabbage	½ cup	2.1
Lettuce (raw)	½ cup	0.8
Sweet Corn, cooked	½ ear	2.4
Legumes		
Beans (baked), canned	⅓ cup	6.2
Peas, frozen, raw,	½ cup	5.7
processed, canned and		
drained	½ cup	5.3
Tomato (fresh)	1 small	1.4
Root Vegetables		
Carrots, young (boiled)	½ cup	2.8
Turnips (raw)	⅔ cup	1.9

* These figures are higher than those for crude fiber usually listed on package labels since the assay method for crude fiber substantially underestimates total dietary fiber.

(Adapted from Southgate, DAT et al: A guide to calculating intakes of dietary fiber. *J. Hum. Nutr.* 30:303, 1976 with permission of the author.)

Food	Portion Size	Total Dietary Fiber/Serving (grams)
Potato—main crops (raw)	one (100 gm)	3.5
—french fries	10 pieces	1.6
—potato chips	3½ ounces	11.9
Fruits		
Apples		
flesh only	1 medium	2.0
peel only	1 medium	0.4
Bananas	1 six inch	1.8
Cherries		
flesh and skin	25 small or 15 large	1.2
Grapefruit, canned, fruit and syrup	½ cup	0.5
Peaches		
flesh and skin	1 medium	2.3
Pear		
flesh only	½ medium	1.1
peel only	½ medium	1.0
Strawberries, raw	10 large	2.1
Nuts		
Peanuts	3½ oz (100 gm)	9.3
Peanut butter	1 tbsp	1.1
Miscellaneous		
Cocoa (beverage)	1 oz	12.1
Strawberry jam	1 tbsp	0.2
Matzoh	1 piece	0.8

an effective way for obese people to lose weight. For the obese diabetic, however, a discussion with a physician should precede an abrupt change to a high-fiber diet, so that weight loss and insulin needs can be carefully watched. At the present time, it seems logical to try more dietary fiber if problems exist such as hemorrhoids, constipation, obesity without diabetes, and diverticulosis.

The table on pages 60–61 shows total dietary fiber by weight in selected foods. It is clear that whole-grain breads and some cereals are high in dietary fiber, raw vegetables are a decent source, and raw fruits contain a fair amount. Note again that canning pears or saucing apples lowers the fiber content by half or more. Conversely, the crude fiber in foods is *less* than the total dietary fiber present, since the chemical method used fails to measure a sizable amount of cellulose and hemicellulose present. Bulk laxatives such as Metamucil basically contain the fiber hemicellulose, the same fiber as in bran cereal and whole-wheat bread, with a gum added that comes from psyllium seeds. Fiber is best thought of as a "natural" laxative and not a nutrient or food supplement.

If you want to try more fiber in your diet, keep the following points in mind:

1. Start with a bran cereal and drink plenty of water with breakfast. Remember that undigested fiber draws water into the bowel, and so the stool is more moist as well as heavier. The water lost in this way must be replaced by drinking more.

2. If bran cereals in milk result in burning diarrhea, the cause is likely lactose intolerance due to failure to digest the milk sugar lactose. In such a situation, switch to bran muffins. A recipe for tasty ones follows this discussion.

3. Fiber after it is eaten will arrive in the colon unchanged, there to be attacked by bacteria. This attack liberates gas, including carbon dioxide and sometimes meth-

ane, and so your constipation may improve but bloating or flatus may increase dramatically for a few days.

4. If your bowel problem is apparent colon disease with either constipation or alternating constipation and diarrhea, try increasing the amount of fiber in the diet *slowly*. For example, a ¾ cup serving of Rice Krispies contains about one gram of total dietary fiber; ¾ cup of cornflakes contains two grams; and ¾ cup of All Bran contains more than eleven grams. A slice of whole-wheat bread contains 1.95 grams of total fiber; a slice of white bread contains but 0.63 gram. It seems prudent to change your brand of cereal *or* the type of bread you eat, at least to start.

5. Hemorrhoid sufferers can really benefit from fiber since the resulting increase in fat and moisture eases the passage when bowel movements occur.

6. Fiber may be useful to *prevent* attacks of diverticulitis. Once pain, fever, or diarrhea starts, however, call a physician and don't take anything by mouth except liquids. For patients with peptic ulcer, there's not enough evidence either to recommend or condemn increased fiber in the diet.

7. For management of simple constipation, fiber should be considered as a bulk laxative at least as effective and clearly safer than stimulant laxatives or soapy enemas.

8. There is no good evidence yet that more fiber prevents heart disease or cancer, or makes for a longer or happier life. The pendulum of opinion on fiber, as with so many other things, tends to reach extremes in either direction, and the present ebullience about the benefits of fiber is likely to subside.

Lou Leibowitz's Best Bran Muffins Ever
as told to her by her mother

7	cups bran
1	box raisins (2½ cups)
2	cups boiling water
1	cup honey
1	cup corn oil
1½	cups molasses (12 oz. jar)
4	eggs, beaten
1	quart buttermilk
3	cups whole-wheat flour (½ cup soy flour may be substituted for part of flour to increase protein content)
5	teaspoons baking soda
1	teaspoon salt

Optional additions: Nuts, dates, crushed pineapple, coconut.

1. Place 4 cups of bran and raisins in a bowl and pour boiling water over. Stir and set aside to cool.
2. Put honey in large bowl and stir in one at a time: oil, molasses, eggs, buttermilk, and remaining 3 cups of bran.
3. Combine flour, soda, and salt. Add to second bran mixture.
4. Stir in bran-raisin mixture.
5. Spoon into greased muffin pans—fill two-thirds full.
6. Bake in preheated 400° F. oven for 20 minutes or till lightly browned.
7. Allow to cool slightly in pan, on racks.
8. Muffins come out more easily if given a short rest period.

Notes: Batter stores in refrigerator, if covered, for up to two months. Bring batter to room temperature before baking.
Muffins freeze well.
Recipe makes approximately 4 dozen muffins of 150 calories each.

5
Gas

A recent television advertisement promised relief from "gasid" indigestion. Gas is not a new medical problem. Some twenty-three centuries ago, Hippocrates, the Greek father of medicine, heard so many complaints about gas from his patients that he wrote his ideas and speculations about the problem in a treatise called "The Winds." The Emperor Claudius repealed laws enacted by the Roman Senate that prohibited the release of gas in public places.

We now know more about intestinal gas than either Hippocrates or Claudius, but as late as 1960 doctors considered spasms of gas—whether belched or passed from the rectum—as not totally explainable if entirely natural events. Several scientists have recently established their reputations and added enormously to our knowledge by measuring gas in various parts of the human intestine. They devised ingenious tubes and passed them into the stomachs, small bowels, or colons of volunteers or desperate patients. Samples of gas can be accurately measured as to amount and chemical composition. As a result, we now know something about what gases exist in the intestine, how they got there, what foods increase gas and why, and what to do to alleviate some common problems. A few myths and recently discovered facts that dispel them are listed in the boxed material on pages 68–69.

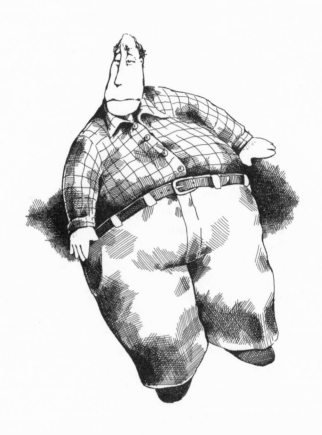

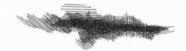

For those who complain of constant belching, bloating, or excessive flatus, gas is a medical condition that deserves thoughtful evaluation and sympathetic management. Bloating is a visible example of gas just as belching and flatus are audible expressions of the symptom. Since belchers, bloaters, and gas passers sound variations on the theme of too much gas, yet complain of quite different sensations and seek relief in different ways, each problem deserves a separate discussion.

The Belcher

If you drink a can of beer or soda, the belches that follow simply represent the release of carbon dioxide that entered your stomach in the liquid you drank. Many of us swallow some air with any food, solid or liquid, and the oxygen and nitrogen have to be released as well. Then too, some foods contain gas—the apple you had with lunch holds 20 percent gas, which must pass one way or the other. We all belch occasionally. The experts who examine chronic belchers often note an upward movement of the Adam's apple as the belcher gulps air in, just before the next belch. With the modern technique of continuous x-ray (fluoroscopy), a chronic belcher can be seen to force air into his esophagus, and nearly all this air is immediately and noisily released back into the atmosphere. The small fraction of the swallowed air not belched out will pass into the stomach. For belchers unwilling to believe this, a sample of the gas in the stomach can be analyzed and yields oxygen, nitrogen, main components of the atmosphere, and a tiny amount of carbon dioxide. It's really swallowed air.

Therefore, chronic belching, especially if the Adam's apple moves up and down during the process, is usually a nervous "gulp and belch" habit. We've all seen cartoons where a character in a dangerous or embarrassing situa-

Myths and Facts about Intestinal Gas

Myths	*Facts*
Since beans, broccoli, and cabbage don't contain gas, they can't be responsible for symptoms of gas.	The foods may be gas free, but each contains complex indigestible sugars broken down by bacteria in the colon to form gas.
"Some days I never pass gas (flatus); other days it never stops."	The average person passes a half liter to two liters of gas a day. Two liters or more are common after eating the foods listed above.
"I don't swallow air, so it must be the damn bacteria."	Probably two-thirds of the gas we belch or pass as flatus was swallowed. Chemical analysis of such gas shows it to have the composition of atmosphere.
"I'm bloated all the time. I bet I have several quarts of gas in my stomach."	At any given time, the gas is in the small intestine, not the stomach, of bloaters, and no more than a cupful is present.

tion will "gulp." Yet many chronic belchers fear that serious underlying conditions such as ulcer or cancer are present. They insist that air swallowing is not the problem, and so this largely self-induced problem is a very difficult one to manage.

The belching process is best understood by watching young infants drink milk. They don't so much sip or drink milk as gulp it. Air is gulped with the milk and the problem of colic (a completely different condition from the similar-sounding "colitis") is due to the inability of infants to belch swallowed air. In some countries where babies are

Myths	Facts
"So my bloating is due to some serious disease!"	Bloating without severe pain or fever is almost never due to disease. Some bloaters have gas that moves more slowly than normal down the intestines.
"I belch constantly. A doctor said I have a hiatus hernia and wants to operate on me."	Most chronic belching is due to excess swallowed air. Of all the symptoms that arise from the bowel (constipation, diarrhea, pain, bleeding, vomiting, weight loss, gas), gas is the symptom *least* likely to reflect a serious health problem.
"I've heard of problems digesting milk, but milk gives me gas more than diarrhea."	Lactose is the sugar in milk that can't be digested by 25% of all adults and can cause either burning diarrhea or, if the lactose is acted on by bacteria, large quantities of gas.

fed while lying on their backs, colic occurs commonly since the milk and air are swallowed and travel down the esophagus, which joins the stomach at the upper *rear* aspect. Therefore, a bubble of gas is often trapped up front as the infant lies on its back. When the bubble cannot be belched, it passes slowly into the small intestine and results in painful colic as the gas causes distension of the wall of the bowel.

The cure—as every mother learns—is to pick up the infant and pat it on the back so that the bubble of swallowed air slowly moves up to a point where it is naturally

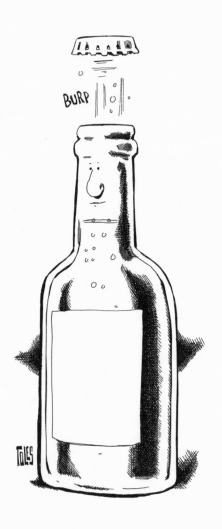

belched out. This longed-for and acceptable belch of mankind brings smiles to all concerned—especially to the fretting baby and its anxious mother. Chronic belchers insist that gulping and then burping air provide temporary relief, but the fluoroscopic x-ray truthfully reveals that more gas is swallowed than is belched out. The problem "inside" cannot be belched out by swallowing air. Nail biters, scratchers, and belchers seem to perpetuate the cycle they themselves have set in motion.

After a heavy meal or a drink or two, women more often than men commonly deal with the pressure sensation of gas by leaning forward slightly and rubbing or gently patting the upper part of their swollen abdomens. Perhaps they recall the technique used to bring relief to the infant distended by gas. Many chronic belchers are treated with drugs that change the function of the stomach or bowels. Now that the origin of belching is clear, such treatment is seen to be obviously irrational and ineffective. Yet, as with so many other forms of "therapy" in medical practice, perhaps the convincing remark "this will work" allows ineffective medicine to bring a sense of relief to some sufferers. As with other common complaints of the gastrointestinal tract—from constipation to hemorrhoids—the chronic belcher deals with his problem through a mixture of lay advice, professional guessing, and trial and error.

Some Suggestions for Belchers

1. Understand that most belches are due to swallowed air, or gas in food. The nervous habit of air swallowing can be broken, and the relief of the belching problem is usually rapid and complete.

2. Holding the mouth slightly open effectively stops belching in some people, since most who gulp air do so with their mouths closed.

3. Chewing gum or sucking on candy helps some people, yet for others, every swallow of saliva delivers more air to the stomach, and sugars often break down to more gas.

4. Simethicone, the active ingredient in products commonly advertised to relieve the "gas" portion of indigestion, may dissolve air bubbles and relieve both belching and bloating. Over-the-counter preparations containing simethicone are safe and relatively inexpensive.

5. Many belchers fail to realize how many carbonated soft drinks they consume. Try water, fruit juice, or skimmed milk instead.

6. Smaller bites of food and slow drinking of fluid usually result in less air swallowed. It's impressive how often the person talking most at mealtime pays least attention to how he eats (and what), and suffers most from belching or bloating after a meal.

7. If, as a chronic belcher, you can find someone who will treat you like a colicky infant, hold you close, pat you gently on the back, and make appropriately soothing sounds after that heavy meal or those delicious drinks, you may consider yourself fortunate indeed, although most adults would prefer to handle their belching problems in a different way.

The Bloater

Most bloaters are men, nearly all are overweight, and they share the conviction that they possess a massive excess of intestinal gas. They can often identify the exact food that "turns to gas" in their bowels, yet for most of these foods no chemical reaction known can explain why eating them should result in gas.

Some bloaters are air swallowers who bloat rather than belch, and when they pay attention to swallowing without gulping air, relief quickly follows. Others are simply too fat, and their adipose tissue is thickened even further by beer that contains grains and sugars that produce both gas and calories, or soda pop bottled with carbon dioxide as part of the manufacturing process. Carbonated beverages with or without calories cause bloating as the gas remains as a bubble in the stomach or passes into the small bowel and distends the wall.

In the last few years, some bloaters have consented to swallow tubes coaxed through the pylorus into the first part of the small intestine—the duodenum—by expert gastroenterologists. A gas foreign to the bowel is pumped in as a kind of marker and all the "native" intestinal gas is flushed out and fastidiously collected at the rectum. Subsequent burps are also collected and the gas is measured. These experiments have shown that both normal subjects and bloated patients have the same volume of gas in the small bowel—at a given moment—only about one cupful! An x-ray study confirms the experiment. Virtually all bloated patients have completely normal volumes of gas in the intestine. The amount present would not fill a balloon larger than an orange. One expert working on this problem reports that this fact is so hard for bloaters to accept— they think a dirigibleful of gas floats inside—that he has the x-ray proof present when he talks to patients.

Another fact may aid understanding. For some bloaters, recent experiments show that, although the *volume* of gas in the small bowel is normal, it moves along very sluggishly and may even paradoxically back up from the small bowel and colon into the stomach again. Normally healthy people will, within fifteen minutes, expel as flatus a gas inserted via a tube into the duodenum. The trip takes no longer than that. In some bloaters, the gas bubble in the bowel simply sits there, or ominously slides in reverse.

Some bloaters also experience rather severe pain with a volume of bowel gas—no more than a cupful, remember—easily tolerated by others. So the bloater may have an "irritable" bowel and therefore feels sensations of uncomfortable fullness or pain that lessens as the belt is loosened. If the motion of gas is sluggish, the "bloat" becomes so much more distressing.

Bloaters often worry about their symptoms until life's last gas is passed, and their demands for relief take on a hostile tone—as though a single, simple cure is available if only doctors would divulge it. That simply isn't true. As with any form of gas that causes symptoms, bloaters will feel better if reassured that no serious disease of the bowels is present.

Since gas passes slowly through the bowels of some bloaters, newly discovered drugs such as metoclopramide may be useful. This drug stimulates smooth muscle, such as that in the wall of the small bowel, and so moves both gas and food along. The drug is sold without a prescription in many countries and is a popular remedy for gas and "indigestion." The Food and Drug Administration in the United States has just approved metoclopramide.

Bloaters who try to get relief with the "swallow and burp" maneuver actually increase the amount of air present and so add to their problem. If they then lie down on their backs after a heavy meal, they will move large bubbles of gas to places in the small bowel where gravity can't work to provide relief, much as happens to milk-fed infants with colic. Available over-the-counter medicines that provide relief for some bloaters include those containing charcoal, which are thought to "absorb gas," simethicone that does seem to break up the gas bubbles, antacids to soothe the bowel, enzymes to cure "maldigestion," and antispasmodic agents that theoretically "relax" the bowel.

Antacids deserve special mention, since many bloaters insist that antacids reduce symptoms. As their name implies, antacids neutralize the effect of hydrochloric acid in the stomach and small bowel. Yet with this neutralizing effect comes the release of a gas—carbon dioxide. Why do bloaters—and belchers for that matter—feel better and not worse if antacids release more carbon dioxide? The answer is that an even greater amount of carbon dioxide is formed when hydrochloric acid reacts with the basic substance bicarbonate normally present in the small bowel. If acid is neutralized by antacids before it meets the bicarbonate, less carbon dioxide is formed. Antacids, therefore, bring relief to some bloated patients.

Simethicone or charcoal may be helpful. A reducing diet for obese bloaters helps both in weight loss and less air swallowing. Moreover, the digestion of fat results in the production of carbon dioxide, an unwanted gas, and so a diet low in fat may work to help in several different ways. And the nap after a heavy meal won't help move the gas. A leisurely walk in place of a rich dessert is a simple and effective suggestion, if a hard one to accept.

Flatus

The human nose can still detect a particularly noxious odor even after the gas has been diluted ten-billionfold so that other sensitive measuring devices record nothing. Not until scientists inserted tubes and meticulously collected rectal gas did newly discovered facts emerge, most as clear as the sound that proclaims their release. Only three gases—carbon dioxide, hydrogen, and methane—are *produced* in the intestine in a quantity large enough to cause symptoms in those with too much gas. Carbon dioxide, the commonest of the three, is not only drunk in sodas and beer, but it bubbles out when hydrochloric acid in the stomach meets bicarbonate in the small bowel, as just discussed for bloaters. Some additional acid is produced as the fat in a meal is digested. A buttery gourmet feast may thus result in the production of several quarts of carbon dioxide. The fullness and bloating sensation that follow a fatty meal may suggest gall-bladder trouble, but the cause is more likely the distension of the stomach and small bowel, both puffed out by carbon dioxide and not food.

To swallow a "bicarb of soda" for relief may make more gas, as this bicarbonate neutralizes additional acid and thus produces more carbon dioxide.

The other two gases formed in the small and large bowel are hydrogen and methane. Hydrogen is the gas that makes balloons lighter than air, and methane is the major constituent in natural gas. Both these gases are produced by the action of bacteria, billions of which multiply constantly in the territory of the small bowel and colon. These bacteria act on sugars that have been taken in the diet and not absorbed, including the milk sugar lactose that one quarter of adults cannot completely digest. The undigested sugars pass into the last part of the small bowel and then into the colon, where bacteria convert them to both hydrogen and carbon dioxide. Bloating, flatus, and diarrhea commonly result. Belching doesn't occur as a symptom because the gas is produced twenty feet further along than the lowest part of the stomach; the small bowel has more turns than a mountain road.

The link between eating baked beans and the passage of massive intestinal gas, especially hydrogen gases, is well known to bean eaters and their dining companions. Bean canners have good reason to support medical research including that carried out at the University of Illinois, where investigators separated beans into several fractions and fed each one separately to normal subjects. The ability of each fraction of bean to produce hydrogen is now specifically known. One fraction is found to contain a large quantity of several sugars (raffinose and other oligosaccharides) that cannot be digested or absorbed, and pass into the colon where the bacteria go to work to produce hydrogen. Some of the hydrogen is released as hydrogen sulfide, which smells like rotten eggs.

Even in forms other than hydrogen sulfide, hydrogen gases stink, and cabbage among other vegetables contains sugars that break down to hydrogen gases. Cabbage is not a fatty food at all, merely a sugary one. Beer bubbles with carbon dioxide, and if the digestive capacity to handle the grain products, malt and hops, is exceeded, foul flatus results. Parties that feature baked beans and beer are best held outdoors.

Some of the gas produced in the intestine ultimately enters the bloodstream and is carried to the lungs and exhaled. If you doubt that gas-blood exchange in the lungs can be rapid, recall that the oxygen that you inhale is partly replaced by carbon dioxide with each breath. The odor of the breath is determined largely by what kinds of gas are produced by bacteria in the colon. Even the pungent odor of the breath imparted by garlic originates most likely not in the mouth but follows the release in the intestine of garlicky gases, which are then carried by the blood to the lungs and exhaled. The characteristic mouth odor of some people presumably reflects the particular strain of bacteria living quietly in their colons. Mouthwash ads omit this fact.

Along with carbon dioxide and hydrogen, the third intestinal gas of man is methane, which is also found in natural gas. Only about one in three adults has intestinal bacteria that produce it. Just as natural gas does, methane burns with a blue flame. Some fraternity boys learn this fact by holding matches close to their blue jeans. The spurt of a blue flame simply confirms that you harbor methane-producing bacteria, not that you are a special form of man. Apparently, if both parents excrete methane, their offspring have a 95 percent chance of being methane producers. A mother confers her own methane-producing bacteria on the fetus before its birth, with persistence for life in the colon of the offspring. Some studies have attempted to link methane production with later cancer of the colon, but the scientific evidence is still fragmentary. And it's really a biologic mystery why two normal subjects can differ in their ability to produce and excrete methane by a factor of 10 million or more.

Most of us, methane excreters or not, pass one or

more types of gas through the sphincter of the anus each day in an amount varying from 250 ml (one cup) to 2 liters. At least one scientist, Dr. Michael Levitt of Minneapolis (who contributed a number of ideas to this chapter), has studied gas passers and belchers so carefully that the editors of the *New England Journal of Medicine*, where his scientific reports appeared, describe him as having conferred "status on flatus" and "class to gas." Dr. Levitt's most famous patient was a twenty-eight-year-old sociology student who had been complaining of excessive gas for about eight years. The student saw a number of doctors, who kept repeating the same x-ray studies of his intestine, diagnosed excessive air swallowing, and tried to counsel him to stop doing it. The student failed to gain relief and decided to scientifically investigate his own problem by keeping a "flatographic" record which indicated frequency of the event and foods eaten. The now-famous student passed gas an average of 34 times a day, about 2½ times normal. When the student drank more milk, he passed more gas. And in 24 hours, he counted a record 141 episodes of flatus.

Dr. Levitt analyzed the gas and found mostly hydrogen, a gas produced in the gut and not present in the atmosphere. Therefore, the specialists were wrong—air swallowing could not have been the cause of his problem. When the student rigorously omitted eating milk sugar (lactose), wheat products, and, of course, beans, the problem subsided almost completely.

If you pass gas excessively—or think you do—the best way to manage it is to determine first if you have an air-swallowing habit. If so, attempt to stop it as outlined for belchers. Then omit the foods, like milk, that may simply not be digested and whose sugars are split into noxious gases by bacteria in the gut. Try omitting beans, cabbage, onions, and wheat products, as well as milk and milk products. If your excessive gas became a problem when you added more fiber to your diet, especially if the high fiber cereal was eaten with milk or the bran muffins were smeared with butter, omit the milk, fiber, and butter in that order and observe the result.

If the match test has proven to you that you excrete methane with your flatus, there is little you can do to eradicate these methane-producing bacteria from your gut. A number of people have learned how to decrease excessive gas by alterations in diet, or by swallowing a favorite antacid or other substance. If it works and isn't dangerous, all well and good. But, of all the ills to which man is heir, excessive gas is perhaps the most embarrassing yet least dangerous.

6
Turista (Traveler's Diarrhea)

Travel expands the mind and loosens the bowels. The result can be called *diarrhea* if bowel movements increase in frequency to two to three times above normal and there is a change in the consistency of the stool from formed to soft or liquid. Defined somewhat more loosely, *diarrhea* describes any bowel movement that fits the shape of the container it is passed into. Since more than 200 million of us travel every year from one country to another, and nearly a quarter of us will develop diarrhea "there," with consequences ranging from a ruined vacation to a decline in tourism as the stories spread, we should learn as much as we can about what traveler's diarrhea or *turista* is due to, and how to prevent or treat it. Those in high office, by the way, are not immune to this disorder—how else can one explain former President Carter's toast to the President of Mexico that included a comment about Montezuma's revenge? Since North American travelers to Mexico number about three million persons per year, and the attack rate of traveler's diarrhea is estimated at 25 to 50 percent, about a million visitors to Mexico return with firsthand experience of the revenge, and many travelers swear off another trip south for just this reason.

The other euphemisms for this problem depend on where you get it. Do you plan on a rendezvous with Ingrid

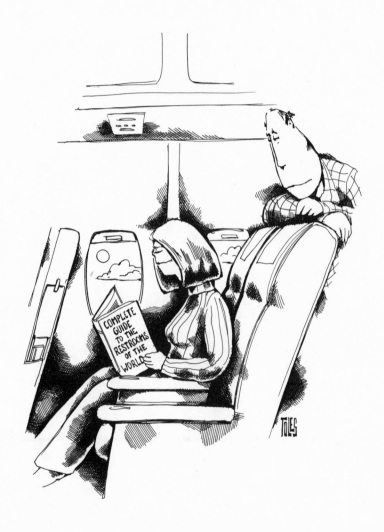

Fact Sheet on *Turista*

Cause
Bacteria eaten or drunk, toxin-producing *E. coli* in 50%; bacteria such as *Salmonella, Shigella* or *Clostridium,* 5% each or less. Viruses in up to 20%. Parasites including *Giardia* in 10%.

Typical attack
On day 5 of the trip, abdominal cramps lead to very watery diarrhea. Appetite is diminished, but vomiting and high fever are *rare*. There are 2 days of severe symptoms and 2 more of mild symptoms. On the 5th day of illness, without treatment save for fluids, the siege is over.

Incriminated foods
1. Fruits and salads
2. Water and milk
3. Foods sold by street vendors

Prevention
1. Avoid incriminated foods.
2. Take Pepto-Bismol, 2 ounces 4 times a day.
3. Take doxycycline if:
   a. A short trip to a high-risk area—Mexico, Peru, El Salvador, India, etc. (see text).
   b. The area has poor medical facilities.
   c. You always get *turista*.
   d. You understand the risks of tetracycline drugs (see text).

in Rick's Café in Casablanca? Don't fall victim to the Casablanca crud. Elsewhere, beware of the Aden gut, the Turkey trot, the Hong Kong dog, the Aztec two-step, or the Delhi belly. A group of Americans who visited Russia developed a form of traveler's diarrhea due to a parasite in the gut called *Giardia lamblia*. The Russians had the

Treatment
1. Fluids. Alternate glasses full of salty or sugary fruit juice, and plain water with baking soda added. You should drink 4 quarts of fluid a day, or more if still thirsty.
2. Lomotil or Imodium; not to exceed 2 tablets 4 times a day in adults; nor for longer than 2 days.

Warnings
1. **Avoid unlabeled anti-diarrhea medicine (see text).**
2. **Stop Doxycycline if *turista* starts while taking it.**
3. **Seek medical help if high fever, black stools, or prolonged vomiting occurs.**

Reassurances
1. Most *turista* is self-limited and cured within a week.
2. *Turista* occurs uncommonly in travelers to Europe and North America.
3. Most *turista* will not require even 24 hours in bed.
4. Replacement of fluid loss is the best therapy.

temerity to suggest that the Leningrad looseness was brought into the country by the visiting Americans. The latter, in turn, coined the term *Trotskys*, a name that has stuck as tightly as the bowels failed to.

The wealthy and fastidious airily comment on the cleanliness of "here" and the dirtiness "there," but travelers visiting cities as clean and prosperous as Geneva may find themselves stricken. And impoverished residents of Calcutta, India, or a small town in Mexico may travel to the United States and be greeted with the "L.A. belly" in southern California or the "Bronxville bomb" in suburban New York. The key ingredient in *turista* is just that—the trip to a new place where one encounters new sights, meets new people, and unwittingly swallows new strains of bacteria.

Unlikely Causes of *Turista*

Many seasoned travelers remain convinced that the anxiety of the trip itself causes the cramps and diarrhea that lay them low in a new environment. This may be true for people who suffer from the variations of normal bowel function referred to elsewhere as apparent colon disease. For those with the gut as a target organ for anxiety, any change from the normal routine may induce diarrhea. The anecdotal travel writers who mention *turista* invoke reasonable but disproven causes, ranging from the stress of travel and sleeplessness to jet lag, overindulgence in alcohol, or the eating of new and "irritating" foods. To combat the stress, some travelers now use tranquilizers such as valium, just as past generations swallowed phenobarbital. Yet *turista* isn't due to stress, and to swallow one valium after another means that when *turista* strikes, the sufferer will calmly stagger rather than rush into the bathroom. As to jet lag, this well-studied condition is related to a physiologic adjustment in many parts of the body, most notably a resetting of the biologic clock, one that requires three to four days to complete. Jet lag may cause the traveler to wake up at unusual hours or fall asleep at the dinner table, and can give rise to mild feelings of disorientation as well as light-headedness and sweating. But *turista* and jet lag are two separate and distinct afflictions of those who travel.

The Overstated Risk of *Turista*

In case you have recently spoken to beleaguered voyagers who describe diarrhea and cramps that incapacitated them during the entire length of the stay in a far-off place, some reassurance before purchasing your own plane ticket is in order. Although *turista* can develop any time one goes from here to there, many areas of the world pose a low risk for travelers. These areas include the British Isles, Scandinavia, most of northern and western Europe, the United States, and Canada. A warm climate, by the way, is not by itself a major factor, since less than one in twelve travelers to Miami or Hawaii has experienced traveler's diarrhea. If you are traveling to visit a relative, and take your meals in private homes, you will very likely avoid diarrhea. The risk is also low with short trips of two or three days, in contrast to a semester's stay at a university abroad; and older people are *less* likely than are the young to develop *turista*. Perhaps they've been exposed to the "cause" enough times to develop resistance or immunity to it. Another reassuring fact is that most *turista* is of mild intensity. A few loose stools may require only minor adjustments in travel plans, and up to half of all travelers who experience *turista* recall little more than their sudden alertness in checking on the location and accessibility of restrooms before starting a meal in a three-star restaurant or a tour through a museum filled with treasures. Less than three of ten travelers afflicted with *turista* have to take to bed because of cramps and weakness. And those who do will feel substantially better within four or five days, even if the only treatment is drinking enough fluids to prevent dehydration.

When are you likeliest to develop *turista?* When you travel to Mexico or certain other Latin American countries, including Peru and El Salvador; Africa, especially Morocco and Kenya; Mediterranean countries, such as Spain and Greece; Middle Eastern countries, including

Iran and Egypt; and Pakistan, India, Bangladesh, and Thailand in the Far East. Surveys have been carried out in each of these countries—unfortunately, the list probably does not end here. *Turista* is likelier to occur in those people who eat in restaurants, and highest in those who succumb to the cries of street vendors, especially if the substance purchased is fruits to be eaten without peeling, fresh vegetables, or ice-cream products already melting before the first bite is taken. In "developing countries" even commercially bottled beverages taken by the wary traveler to assuage thirst and ward off the problem of "impure water" may not be safe—beverages are bottled under varying sanitary conditions.

Why the Problem in Studying *Turista*?

To study *turista* with any hope of learning something requires persuading a group of prospective travelers to provide stool samples before they travel, while they are away, and when they return. Some truly obsessed scientists go *with* the travelers, whether students or soldiers, and set up what amounts to a major bacteriology laboratory in often primitive settings. Try sterilizing glassware in a jungle swamp. As if this were not enough, the travelers being studied have to cooperate fully to remember and give details about each food and how much of it they eat, what liquids they drink, where they go, what they do, and with whom they do it!

Although interviewing travelers thoroughly is a difficult task, the accurate study of the soft stool itself poses an enormous challenge. The chapter on how the bowel works tells that each lump of stool large enough to see contains billions of bacteria. A given bacterium is first grouped according to its genus. A single such genus consists of many bacterial brothers and sisters called species. Species are separated one from another by simple measures, such as noting the color of a bacterial colony, but more complex tests may be necessary, such as the ability to ferment a certain sugar. Then, too, whole genera are called anerobic since they won't grow if even small amounts of oxygen are present. Finally, certain species of bacteria known to cause diarrhea in some people may reside unnoticed in many normal persons. Add these matters to the central one that many bacterial genera live in the rich garden called the flora of the colon, with multiple species in each genus. It's clear why several scientists have suggested that anyone who desires to study human stool from the point of view of the bacterial populations present should be incarcerated for his own benefit until the urge subsides.

Is Anything Really Known?

Yes. In spite of all the problems listed, science has triumphed, after a fashion; it is possible to say with reasonable certainty that the cause of *turista* is one or more strains of bacteria or other types of living creatures (parasites, viruses) that have been swallowed and have taken root in the garden of the small bowel or colon. Some of these organisms have been linked to *turista* for a hundred years or more.

One of them, swallowed in food or water, has caused epidemics of diarrhea for centuries, with death due to dehydration in malnourished infants and adults. This is *V. cholera* (*V.* for the genus *Vibrio*, whose species move in a vibrating manner when viewed under a microscope) and the species that cause cholera produce a toxin that results in a rush of water from tissues into the bowel and then out as diarrhea. Although cholera epidemics probably ravaged civilizations before the Crusades and certainly thereafter (the Death in Venice that established Thomas Mann as a great writer was undoubtedly cholera), cholera is now exceedingly rare as a cause of diarrhea in well-nourished travelers, whether children or adults.

A second genus of bacteria, described by Dr. Daniel

Salmon in the late 1800s, is now called *Salmonella*. The species usually gets its name from the city where it was first isolated, so that outbreaks of *Salmonella heidelberg* or *Salmonella montevideo* or *Salmonella newporti* have occurred. These bacteria are often unknowingly eaten with poorly prepared or undercooked poultry and eggs or drunk as contaminated milk and water, and species of *Salmonella* cause disease that exactly resembles *turista*, with cramps, diarrhea, and little or no fever. One strain of *Salmonella—typhosa—*causes typhoid fever. A few of us, whether travelers or not, may carry *Salmonella* bacteria in the gut or gall bladder without symptoms, and such carriers may unknowingly infect others, as typhoid Mary did. When vomiting, diarrhea, and abdominal cramps afflict hundreds of people who ate the same egg salad at a church picnic or shared the same egg-based dessert at a giant bar mitzvah dinner, one of a hundred or more species of *Salmonella* is one likely cause, among others, for the food poisoning. As a cause of *turista*, though, *Salmonella* is responsible for no more than 10 percent of all cases.

First cousins to *Salmonella* bacteria are those in the genus *Shigella*, which can be transported from uncovered feces to someone else's food by ordinary house flies. That's one reason for campers to dig latrines deep, or cover feces with plenty of earth. Once food is contaminated, those who eat it will enjoy one or two more days of good health and then develop diarrhea alone, diarrhea and crampy belly pain, or both of these with fever. The trouble is usually in the small bowel.

Should *Shigella* infect the wall of the large bowel, and this sometimes occurs, the invaded colon pains and bleeds. This disease is known as bacillary dysentery, a form of true colitis; the afflicted traveler experiences severe cramps and painful urgency, tenesmus, that impels him to race from bed to toilet. The diarrhea may occur as frequently as every fifteen minutes, the scant stool produced is composed primarily of blood and mucus, and the high fever and cramping pain may bring sufferers to their knees. It was this illness that devastated the German troops at El Alamein in North Africa in World War II, although General Bernard Law Montgomery, head of the British Eighth Army, is also accorded credit for the victory. However, most patients with *Shigella* diarrhea do not have blood in the stool and have a disease so mild that someone will ascribe their symptoms to *turista*. As with *Salmonella*, no more than 10 percent of *turista* is caused by strains of *Shigella*.

Another genus of bacteria is *Clostridium*, which can cause food poisoning with diarrhea and cramps, as well as gas gangrene in wounded soldiers. To grow, most strains require the complete absence of oxygen, a condition met in, say, a thick gravy that covers meat in which spores (seedlings) of *Clostridia* await their chance to multiply. Though the fact is hard to believe, gravy initiated a tragic sequence of events that caused the death from *Clostridium* infections of several nursing-home residents in the northeast United States within the last few years. As another example of a clostridium problem, consider the New Guinea highlanders who experienced profound stomach ache and diarrhea accompanying the ritual feasting on undercooked and infected pork. They coined the term *pig bel*, which describes the cause and result very clearly. Diarrhea in starved people being fed was termed *Darmbrand* or "fire in the belly" in Germany at the close of World War II, and the cause was likely *Clostridium*. But *Clostridium* as a cause of *turista?* Probably 2 percent or less.

To prove that a species of *Shigella*, *Salmonella*, or *Clostridium* is the cause of diarrhea, a sample of stool obtained from the patient must be "cultured," which requires growing the bacteria present in the stool in a laboratory under controlled conditions. Only then can the diagnosis be pinpointed. Some of the living things that travelers unknowingly swallow are not bacteria at all but may be creatures called protozoans, including amebas, which cause amebic dysentery. In some parts of the world, where "sanitary" conditions belie the very meaning of the word, amebas abound in food and water, and they are shed in the stools of both sick and apparently well persons. Amebiasis was once considered an important cause of *turista,* and tons of antibiotics, including some dangerous ones, were prescribed to eradicate the amebas. The short-term visitor to areas where amebiasis is common runs small risk of amebic dysentery, and most experts feel that, as a cause of *turista,* amebiasis is even *less* common than *Shigella, Salmonella,* or *Clostridium.* Another protozoan, *Giardia lamblia,* was the cause of the "Trotskys" that afflicted the travelers to Leningrad. Although *Giardia* are responsible for only about 2 percent of *turista,* they cause a true malabsorption of fat, and those afflicted will complain not only of diarrhea but weight loss and greasy stools as well. Giardiasis usually results from drinking the cysts, the "unsprouted seeds" of the protozoans, and these cysts have been recovered from drinking water that caused infection in campers in Utah; in the citizens of Rome, New York; Bradford, Pennsylvania; and Washington state. In all the outbreaks, the water supply was contaminated. These *Giardia* are successfully wiped out when patients are given the drug metronidazole (Flagyl).

The Percentages Don't Add Up

The subject is clearly a complex one, which is why a single approach to prevention or treatment of *turista* won't work. For example, viruses, which are living creatures much smaller than bacteria, can cause diarrhea; and parasites, including hookworm and many others, do the same. Even new genera of bacteria are being discovered that are implicated in some people with *turista,* including species of the recently discovered genera of *Campylobacter* and *Yersinia*. So the stool from a traveler afflicted with *turista* can be investigated for every living thing present—at which point the traveler will have returned home some weeks before—and still, in about one half the cases, no likely cause is apparent.

Any Other Explanations?

Yes, and it took years to find the answer. In the teeming population of the gut, the commonest bacteria that use oxygen are strains of *Escherichia coli*, a species so prominent that every stool sample from whatever source can be coaxed to yield several strains of *E. coli*. Research in the last ten years proves that a number of perfectly innocuous-appearing *E. coli* may produce a toxin—a poison, really—that attacks the wall of the small bowel and causes it to secrete fluid and salts as diarrhea. *It is now clear that a third to a half of all cases of* turista *are caused by these toxin-producing E. coli bacteria.* This secret was unearthed only after diligent research over many years. The reason for the delay, among others, is that a toxin-producing *E. coli* strain looks like any other in a culture unless complex tests in experimental animals are done to prove that a toxin really exists.

So we can now say with some certainty that *turista* is due to one of several bacteria or other living organisms, most likely a toxin-producing *E. coli*, that we have eaten or drunk while traveling. Somehow, these organisms new to us have found or made a place in the intestine, have multiplied there, and now either inflame the wall of the large bowel directly or produce a toxin that does so. Thus the *E. coli* may have been swallowed on the second day of the trip, their number doubling every thirty minutes, and now, forty-eight hours later, the illness begins. For some travelers, it is merely a loosening of the stool and increase in number of bowel movements. In others, the severe cramps, nausea, and profound diarrhea render the fevered traveler truly delirious for home. For most of the afflicted, the illness will subside *by itself* in four days, two of unpleasant diarrhea and two of gradual improvement.

How Can I Prevent *Turista*?

If there were a single answer, we would not need thousands of words to tell about it and boards of tourism could cease worrying. Keep in mind that the following comments refer to prevention of *turista* before it begins, not treatment once you've got it.

1. *Show caution.* The first point to make about prevention is that in high-risk areas one should avoid tap water, ice cubes, salads, unwashed fruits and vegetables, custards and cream desserts, unpasteurized milk and dairy products, and all items offered by street vendors. Be constantly alert. Don't spurn tap water and then brush your teeth with it, or swallow your sleeping pill with a glassful. And can you avoid ice cubes when you've been handed a warm gin and tonic in 100-degree heat? The thirsty traveler can try to rely on bottled water and canned and bottled beverages, but, as we said before, local bottling conditions vary. Even the most fastidious traveler can be plagued by an outbreak of *turista.*

2. *A warning.* A drug of reputed value in prevention or treatment of *turista*, its worth passed on by word of mouth by successive generations of international travelers, was the drug iodochlorhydroxyquin (Enterovioform). DON'T TAKE THIS DRUG OR ALLOW IT TO BE SOLD TO YOU. First of all, it doesn't work in either preventing or treating *turista*. More important, this drug is associated with damage to the nervous system, including blindness. Forget about Enterovioform, and throw away any that still gathers dust in the medicine cabinet. The sale of the drug is

forbidden in the United States, but it is available elsewhere.

3. *Bismuth.* The old-time remedy Pepto-Bismol contains the bismuth salt that was touted to travelers for more than a century without any proof that it really worked. Yet, when students traveling to Mexico recently took Pepto-Bismol as a preventive agent, *before* diarrhea began, those who swigged the pink liquid in a dose of two ounces four times a day had a 23 percent rate of diarrhea, whereas the untreated students had a 61 percent rate. If you're going to be away for two weeks, you will have to pack well over a hundred ounces of Pepto-Bismol and some customs official may give you a meticulous going-over upon uncovering those rows of bottles. Keep in mind that, even with high doses of this agent, more than a fifth of the students who came to Mexico still experienced *turista.* Unless you get nauseated from looking at the pink color, the medicine is certainly safe.

4. *Doxycyclines.* The most promising antibiotic to *prevent* or protect against *turista* is a long-acting tetracycline drug called doxycycline (Vibramycin). Some very good studies including one among American Peace Corps volunteers in Kenya and another in Morocco showed that the drug worked to prevent *turista* in 90 percent of the Peace Corps volunteers at risk. This antibiotic works as a preventive measure by eradicating toxin-producing *E. coli* before these bacteria multiply in the bowel to cause *turista.* And the drug is relatively safe, certainly more so than the dangerous Enterovioform or concoctions sold on the street.

Yet most experts in infectious diseases would *not* take doxycycline for prevention of *turista.* The reasons they give are borne out by recent medical evidence:

1. Doxycycline belongs to the tetracycline family of antibiotics. Some agents in this group can damage the fetus and should not be used by pregnant women. Many of them may cause permanent staining and other damage to

unerupted teeth, so, to be on the safe side, children under age eight should not take these drugs. Some tetracycline drugs cause a greatly heightened sensitivity to sunlight, which may in turn produce severe skin rashes.

2. Doxycycline is a broad-spectrum antibiotic that will eradicate billions of bacteria that normally live and multiply in the bowel. They may therefore clear the way for disease-producing bacteria to multiply in comfort, especially a bacterial species resistant to doxycycline. Such bacteria include strains of *Shigella* and *Salmonella* (themselves causes of some *turista*); as well as some strains of toxin-producing *E. coli* that happen to be natively resistant to the drug. Yeast infections may also occur, especially in women taking birth-control pills.

3. Doxycycline causes nausea, vomiting, diarrhea, or dizziness in some patients.

For these reasons, the advisory memorandum on traveler's diarrhea published by the Center for Disease Control in Atlanta in January 1980 states: "We do not have enough information on risks and benefits of use of doxycycline for preventing diarrhea to make general recommendations for travelers." Several experts consulted on the *prevention* of *turista* suggested dietary restraint and perhaps the use of Pepto-Bismol. Doxycycline may be considered for travelers going to high-risk areas for short-term visits of fourteen days or less; for experienced travelers who invariably get *turista;* and for those planning brief stays during which they require uninterrupted use of their time for business or professional purposes. For the casual vacationer, doxycycline cannot be given an endorsement.

Treatment of *Turista*

By the time you read this chapter, you may be well past the prevention stage and need treatment for diarrhea and/or cramps. The following points are useful:

1. You will feel somewhat better and avoid dangerous dehydration if you drink enough *fluids*, especially
those containing sugar and salts. Alternating glasses of
fruit juice, with added salt and sugar, and water containing ¼ teaspoon of baking soda per glass can replace the
fluid, sugar, and salt lost with *turista*. Be careful about
drinking too much Coca-Cola or coffee, since the caffeine
will increase the motility of the colon. Alcohol has a similar effect. Milk and dairy products are best avoided.

2. Of the nonspecific remedies, hundreds of *anti-
diarrhea nostrums* can be found in locations ranging from
pharmacies to soothsayers' booths. In many countries of
the world, labeling requirements are very lax, and *the
traveler with* turista *may therefore be swallowing a concoction of drugs, sold on the street or over the counter,
that contains potentially dangerous medicine*. Two common ones are the antibiotic chloramphenicol, which can
damage the bone marrow with fatal results, and Enterovioform, which can cause loss of vision. It thus makes
sense to avoid all anti-diarrhea medicine sold in other
countries unless a label of ingredients is present and can
be inspected.

3. The British favor the use of morphine added to
either chalk or kaolin, but the amount of narcotic is too
low for either a euphoric high or a colonic slow. Kaopec-
tate contains kaolin, pectin, and hydrate aluminum sili-
cate. The combination is supposed to absorb water and
thus convert liquid diarrhea into mush. This has little effect in controlling diarrhea. Eating yogurt is even less effective for this purpose. Some people believe eating yogurt
alters the balance between the good lactobacilli and the
bad *E. coli*. In fact, however, the only positive medical
value of eating yogurt is that it satisfies hunger.

4. A number of marketed drugs *reduce the motility
of the bowel*. Most of them are related to opium-type
drugs but have been chemically altered to slow down the
gut without landing you in jail for behaving strangely on

the street. *Paregoric* has been swallowed for over a century, and works fairly well. In a dose of one or two teaspoons after each loose stool, not to exceed four times a day, paregoric works, although experienced observers describe a distinctly "high" feeling from the tincture of opium in paregoric, which a few of them welcome as they wait out the ravages of *turista*.

A variant of the powerful drug Demerol (meperidine) is diphenoxylate, or *Lomotil*, which is usually prepared with a small amount of atropine to prevent abuse. One or two tablets can be taken every six hours until diarrhea is controlled. If simple *turista* is not improved within a twenty-four-hour period—with up to eight tablets of Lomotil, for example—do not use the drug further. A newer drug resembling Lomotil, Imodium (loperamide), can be taken in four-milligram doses (two tablets), followed by two milligrams (one tablet) after each unformed stool—not to exceed eight tablets a day in an adult. These agents should be avoided by pregnant women and especially young children, in whom signs of narcotic overdose may be seen. Caution is advised for travelers who take tranquilizers, sedatives, or alcohol; Lomotil is a synthetic narcotic. Ask your doctor about possible drug interactions.

Lomotil or related anti-motility drugs are relatively safe and rather effective, although there is no convincing proof that these drugs reduce the total amount of water released in the stool. Quite often, a few tablets of Lomotil or Imodium will cause symptoms to abate. Remember that any drug that slows the motility of the colon, and all of these agents do just that, may allow the additional growth of the very *E. coli* that are incriminated as a cause of *turista*. Thus the observed paradox wherein the *turista* sufferer who takes pills feels better with less diarrhea, but his symptoms last twice as long as those of a traveling companion who merely reduces activity and drinks plenty of fluids. If *high fever* develops or the stools are bloody, avoid all of these drugs and seek the best medical help available.

5. Finally a word about using *antibiotics* to treat *turista*, not prevent it. The list of causes of *turista* is long, and many of the causative organisms will not be eradicated by small doses of antibiotics. Keep in mind that the *turista* will likely subside within four to five days, and if symptoms persist after that time, a stool culture should be obtained. If the cause is *Salmonella* or *Shigella* or *Clostridium* or *Giardia*, each requires therapy with a different antibiotic. Doxycycline is valuable in preventing *E. coli*-caused *turista*, but its value in treating the disease is as yet unproven. In many countries outside the United States, anti-diarrhea medicine may contain several antibiotics aside from the dangerous one, chloramphenicol.

In a strange land, racked with cramps and diarrhea, the traveler may eagerly swallow the unlabeled concoction sold over the counter, but as we have discussed, such "cures" may be far worse than the disease itself. Replacement of lost fluid and salt and a few days of rest comprise the most effective therapy.

7
Hemorrhoids (Piles)

The human anus is much more than a simple hole. Only an inch long, the anal canal and its purse-string sphincter hold the contents of the rectum in place hour after hour, opening only when a major muscle contraction of the lower colon commands them to do so. The examining physician who "does a rectal" starts by looking at the anus for hemorrhoids and many other disorders, such as skin infections and pinworms (which can cause itching), anal fissures (sore breaks in the anal lining), fistulas, cancer, venereal diseases, and simple injuries. As for the last, anything one can imagine and more has been inserted through the rectal sphincter and into the canal.

Normal passage of formed stool requires that muscular contractions of the colon be finely coordinated with opening of the anal sphincter. The colon contractions propel the stool along with motions that are described in Chapter 2, How the Bowel Works. These motions have mysterious origins but they clearly cannot be willed into existence. To force defecation by bearing down is a useless, unrewarding exercise that leads to anal problems. One such price paid for straining at stool is the development of hemorrhoids, otherwise known as "piles," that are subject to pain, bleeding, and other discomforts. Yet millions of adults suffer from piles even though they don't strain at stool, haven't borne children, and don't complain of chronic constipation. So several questions can be asked: What causes hemorrhoids? What are they? And why do some hemorrhoids bleed, hurt, or prolapse (fall out of place and fail to return) while many others bring their owners no difficulties whatever?

Herewith some partial answers. Although our four-legged ancestors and present-day pets go through life unencumbered by hemorrhoids, piles likely annoyed the first human being who assumed an upright stature. *Half or more of the adult population possess them,* although symptoms are often trivial or absent altogether. Yet hemorrhoids are so commonly found that it may be abnormal *not* to have them, a small consolation for the afflicted. In general, women and men suffer in equal numbers. One interesting point is that persons with primarily sedentary jobs are *not* more subject to hemorrhoids than are physically active workmen. Piles are often the first tangible lump to appear on the person of a pregnant woman and are no less a harbinger of the coming blessed event than is breast tenderness or morning nausea.

Hemorrhoids are composed of blood vessels that form into mounds or piles as the loose, movable inner lining of the anal canal works its way out through the anus. The big veins in this lining become unwillingly trapped, stranded outside by the tight muscle of the anal sphincter that won't allow re-entry. To envision how the inner lining of the anus gets stuck outside short of everything else breaking loose, imagine the following: A well-dressed man in blazer and white shirt drops his subway token into a hole three feet deep. In order to retrieve the coin he kneels beside the hole and reaches in, but is not quite able to touch bottom. At this point his shirt cuff is far out of the blazer sleeve—an excellent example of a lining dropping from its proper position, as does that of the anal canal. After the final stretch for the last inch needed to grasp the coin, the man stands up, only to find his coat sleeve bunched up near his elbow in a fixed position, while the shirt cuff remains outside. This situation, if not corrected with the other hand or by vigorous shaking, may persist.

In the anal canal a moist version of a similar event takes place and causes entrapment of anal veins outside the rectum and their subsequent enlargement into hemorrhoids. The lining of the anus is criss-crossed by big veins as fat as those on the back of the hand; when these become trapped by the muscular purse string of the anus, the veins can't drain their blood and gradually or suddenly enlarge to the size of cherries or plums. If you happen to notice such an enlarging lump, the trapped vessels can be gently pushed back in where they belong. This maneuver is a simple one for all but the most fastidious individuals and is made entirely antiseptic when done with a rubber glove or finger cot (obtainable at the drugstore) placed on the deployed digit. Since the blood vessels in the lump are fragile, injured, and misplaced, the need for gentleness is obvious.

The force that pushes out the anal lining and its veins is pressure from above that comes about by the squeezing of abdominal muscles during defecation. The intensity of this effort is apparent to all who have been seated in a toilet stall within earshot of their grunting and constipated fellow man. The muscular effort causes veins to bulge fore and aft. Because the colon and rectum have failed to generate a smooth and strong coordinated action, such constipated and determined people try to force stool past the closed anus, an effort doomed to failure at stool but success at sprouting hemorrhoids. Defecation requires rhythmic smooth-muscle action in the colon wall and is in no way aided by rigorous tensing of abdominal muscles. Small wonder that the anal lining finally loses its grip.

Well, then, why is it that people without constipation who aren't pregnant and don't bear down mightily while seated in the bathroom still develop hemorrhoids? There's no clear consensus among experts. However, a day or two of diarrhea may trigger the development of hemorrhoids or set off a startling attack of hemorrhoid pain or prolapse in someone who hitherto has lived in harmony with his or her affliction. But all theories on why this condition occurs at all are highly suspect and not very illuminating. In truth, the cause of hemorrhoids remains a mystery, but straining at stool plays a major role in most cases.

Piles may go unnoticed but more typically draw attention to themselves from time to time. There are three major symptoms—itching, pain, and bleeding. Hemorrhoids hurt terribly when the blood inside suddenly clots and in so doing tugs on the wall of the vein. The pain of such a thrombosed hemorrhoid lasts for several minutes to as long as an hour and can be compared to having a sharp nail pushed steadily against the wall of the anus. This unique sensation typically begins without warning and will stop any but the most absorbing conversation in midsentence. These attacks may be relatively mild or incapacitating and may occur several times a day for a cluster of days, only to disappear until they return for another round weeks, months, or even years later.

During the acute stages the hemorrhoids are bulging, shiny, and sore, but the clotting event typically damages the cherry-sized mass to such an extent that it shrivels into a dense lump, much smaller than its former self, one that the doctor calls a hemorrhoidal tag. These tags are wrinkled monuments on the battlefield of past hemorrhoidal pain. Hemorrhoids can also hurt, with lesser intensity, if rubbed too hard by bargain-basement toilet paper of the type prized by purchasing agents for schools, hospitals, and other marginally solvent institutions. No one can predict or escape a siege of hemorrhoidal pain—both George Brett, third baseman for the Kansas City Royals in the 1980 World Series, and former President Jimmy Carter suffered hemorrhoid problems as well as national publicity about their ailment. Severe hemorrhoidal pain not relieved in a matter of days usually leads the sufferer to a doctor who can provide instant relief by cutting open the vein and removing the clot. This is a minor procedure *very different* from a formal hemorrhoidectomy, although the brief surgical encounter is conducted on a special table that places the patient in the undignified posture of having the anus firmly positioned in mid-air.

Anal itching is a related problem well known to the man on the street even if, by chance, he has an anus which has managed to escape the curse of hemorrhoids. Who can drive from the mind the brilliant capstone of the advertising copywriter's art: "The torment of rectal itch"? The line is masterly in its ability to convert a minor annoyance into a major evil that persuades one to purchase relief. Anal itching, like all other itching, is simply a mild variant of pain, as the nerves which convey pain sensation also handle itching and burning. Because these symptoms are less troublesome but more chronic than is the sudden severe pain of thrombosis, careful attention is needed to protect piles from long-standing physical abuse caused by repeated wiping, scratching, and probing. This is not a simple matter, as hemorrhoids reside in a dark, moist place in constant contact with bacteria-filled stool, some of which is rubbed into already inflamed tissue with every bit of toilet paper. These unpleasant facts require understanding so that a rational approach to hemorrhoid symptoms can be undertaken.

Coping with Hemorrhoids

Anal Hygiene. First and foremost, handle this aching region gently. It is very important to keep hemorrhoids clean. Not *wiped* clean, but *washed* clean! Gently *pat* the itching hemorrhoid clean rather than using a brisk rub with pressure that gives surcease for seconds while ensuring further tissue inflammation and symptoms for days. Soothe inflamed tissue by patting softly with toilet paper moistened in warm water. When the anus is clean, apply plenty of baby powder to maintain dryness and to allow tissues to move freely among one another.

Sitz Baths. After a bowel movement, with the anus patted clean, the next step is simple but crucial. The itching and soreness of piles often yield to that greatest of healers, hot water, a therapeutic agent of such low cost and ready availability that it is the treatment *least* likely to come to mind. *Why* hot water works is unknown. Relief, however, awaits the diligent man or woman who places the posterior in very hot water for fifteen minutes after every bowel movement or twice daily. This time-honored maneuver is known as the *sitz bath,* from the German word "to sit." Because a sitz bath requires only a tub, hot water, and a sore rear end, even the suggestion that it works evokes a great deal of unwarranted skepticism. After all, one may argue, how can hot water unfortified with costly medication possess curative properties? One indoctrinated soul added bouillon cubes to the hot bathing liquid and has since claimed that chicken soup heals hemorrhoids!

Be as skeptical as you will, but sitz baths work. To modify the procedure, place a large flat rock in the water. This brings the hot water to a higher level. Many pharmacies sell "sitz baths," plastic seats that fit on an opened toilet. A most important detail when "sitzing" is to avoid burning oneself, although the hotter the water, the better. In order to prevent injury to the skin this treatment should be used no more than twice a day for a week. By that time symptoms should be gone anyway. Remember to pat the heated anus dry when the sitz is over, and add powder liberally.

Bleeding. Piles frequently bleed. For the same reason that all the juice doesn't pour out of a hole poked into an orange, piles don't bleed heavily because they have a honeycombed interior whose chambers bleed in short bursts, a few at a time. Bleeding may announce itself as a streak of red blood on the stool or toilet paper. Such bleeding must always be taken seriously because anemia may result if bleeding is heavy or of long duration. A greater danger from bleeding is that it is ascribed to hemorrhoids and thus draws attention away from a far more serious disease of the bowel, namely colon cancer. Sad to say, many patients ignore rectal bleeding in the mistaken or hopeful belief that the blood comes from piles rather than cancer. Because early detection of colon cancer makes treatment easier and more effective, *every person who bleeds from the rectum or anus, in any amount, must be examined by a doctor.* Nine times out of ten it will be the piles that are bleeding, but there is no reason to gamble with your own health at stake.

If you tell your doctor you saw blood in the stool or on the toilet paper and he or she fails to do a complete rectal examination, find another doctor. The full investigation of bleeding from below must involve the insertion of a sigmoidoscope, an instrument through which the doctor can view up to 20 cm of the anal canal, rectum, and lower colon. X-rays of the bowel are often needed as well. Bleeding can be correctly attributed to piles only when other disorders have been excluded, and a prudent physician will always assume that rectal bleeding in adults suggests cancer until proven otherwise. These proper examinations may save your life, as the section on cancer of the colon describes (see page 119).

Surgery. A few hemorrhoid sufferers experience many large and uncomfortable hemorrhoids over months or years which refuse to yield to sitz baths, improved bowel habits, powders, sitting on doughnut pillows, and perhaps an astringent ointment that shrinks tissue as do nosedrops elsewhere. A patient having such prolonged misery probably needs surgical attention in the form of a hemorrhoidectomy. This operation is offered frequently but should not be agreed to casually. Be sure you have a highly qualified specialist—inept surgery can damage the anal canal and result in a scar or stricture that will compound the original problem. A less dramatic but troublesome matter that follows one in ten major hemorrhoid operations is the inability of the patient to distinguish gas from stool, the nerves gathering this crucial information having been damaged during rectal surgery. Indeed, it is the fine neurological tuning of the normal rectum as well as a very useful awareness that allows us to differentiate two similar sensations. With all these caveats in mind, major hemorrhoid surgery (not the incision to drain a single clotted hemorrhoid) is clearly necessary in only a few pile sufferers. The operation requires an expert surgeon, preferably a proctologist who specializes in these matters. It is prudent to ask for a second opinion before the cutting starts, especially if hemorrhoid symptoms are infrequent or began recently.

Once surgery becomes an unavoidable alternative, another problem arises: What kind of surgery should be done? Traditionally all the veins are removed in the lower rectum, the logic being that veins no longer present can't bubble into future hemorrhoids. A lesser procedure is injection of the piles with chemicals that induce intensive inflammation that causes the veins to become scarred and shriveled when they heal. This approach is a first cousin of the procedure once popular for the surgical treatment of varicose veins in the legs. Two other surgical procedures have recently been developed and they show promise. The first involves tying off the enlarged veins with a rubber band skillfully wrapped around the base of the hemorrhoid under view of a proctoscope. Because this procedure chokes off the blood supply, the venous tumor has no alternative but to die and dissolve over the ensuing week or two, cleanly and quietly. The technique is somewhat painful but so effective that the patient forgets the few days of discomfort as months pass without recurrent rectal symptoms.

A second technique recently reported from Britain is

the Lord procedure, in which the anal opening is forcibly enlarged to allow the anal lining and its big veins the opportunity to slide back up where they belong. This operation is successful presumably because the single most important problem leading to hemorrhoids may be an abnormally tight anus. As mentioned earlier, the tightness of the anal muscle (sphincter) will not allow the veins and tissues which have crept out during the forward surge of a bowel movement to later crawl back in. The enlargement of the anus in the Lord technique is designed to *weaken* the abnormally strong sphincter, and although the operation would seem to expose the patient to the risk of leaky anus later on, such problems usually do not occur. The procedure is named after the physician who described it. The Lord dilatation maneuver requires the insertion into the rectum of four fingers of both the surgeon's hands simultaneously. For obvious reasons, this operation requires general anesthesia. Shortly after surgery, the anus closes again to its proper size.

Summary. So hemorrhoids may be cut out, strangled with a rubber band, swept up a dilated sphincter, shriveled by sclerosing chemicals, and, with the advent of cryosurgery, can even be frozen to death. And, having tolerated one or more of these violent-sounding "cures," the patient may be free of symptoms for a while, only to discover another characteristic of hemorrhoids: they recur. It's enough to send most people with minor or infrequent hemorrhoid problems to their simple sitz bath of hot water.

The subject of high-fiber diets and bulkier stool is discussed in detail elsewhere. More fiber in the diet results in easier passage of better-lubricated stool, an ideal situation for those with painful or itching hemorrhoids. And, finally, what of astringents, such as Preparation H, sold as ointments or in suppository form? Astringents shrink swollen anal tissue and are suitable for occasional use for relief of hemorrhoidal pain and itching, but chronic use has been

shown to diminish their effect. Most flareups of hemorrhoidal symptoms will respond fully to twice-a-day sitz
baths in quite hot water, with liberal use of powder when
the rear has been patted dry, and perhaps Preparation H
ointment inserted morning and night. Except for fiber or
stool softeners, laxatives should be avoided during acute
attacks of hemorrhoids. The best defense against hemorrhoids is a normal bowel habit, but even regularity and
bulk afford no sure protection for the anus.

It is worth emphasizing that rectal bleeding requires
thoughtful investigation by a physician who won't prema-
turely ascribe blood to hemorrhoids, *even if bleeding
hemorrhoids are present,* until more serious diseases of the
colon and rectum, namely cancer and ulcerative colitis,
are ruled out. And when they are—and the fear of serious
illness dissolves—eat bran muffins with plenty of water,
stay away from the "hemorrhoid doctor" who repeatedly
advises rectal surgery, sit in very hot water, and comfort
yourself with the knowledge that thousands of others are
healing their hemorrhoids in exactly the same way.

HB 1 M

8
Three Serious Diseases of the Colon

Not all colon problems are trivial or self-limited. Of the topics discussed so far, excess gas doesn't hurt anyone, hemorrhoids heal with hot water, *turista* is a temporary condition, bran and other dietary fiber can take the place of harsh contact laxatives and enemas, most colon pain and constipation are not due to colon disease after all, and the large bowel isn't even required for digestion of nutrients to occur. Much of this comes as good news to people genuinely worried about symptoms. Yet it is also true that serious disease of the colon is diagnosed daily in hundreds of hitherto healthy and so unprepared young people and adults. Three such common diseases of the colon must be discussed in detail: diverticulitis, ulcerative colitis, and cancer of the colon. Each of them occurs often, can be diagnosed precisely, and responds to proper therapy. Any informed physician who carefully questions and examines patients can manage these diseases, although a hospital admission is usually required for thorough evaluation, and expert consultants are often called in to help.

This book is not a guide to self-treatment of colon disease, a comment worth emphasizing. The purpose of this chapter, and that of the entire book, in fact, is to make you aware of the normal functioning of the colon and how it can go awry. But the assessment of symptoms requires an expert. Proper diagnosis and therapy of all illnesses of the bowel, real or apparent, call for careful attention to *your* complaints by *your* doctor. It is undeniable that most diarrhea without blood is self-limited and of little importance, yet diarrhea is the commonest symptom of ulcerative colitis. Rectal bleeding usually results from hemorrhoids, a minor problem; but some episodes of bleeding announce the presence of diverticulitis or cancer of the colon. Whether your symptoms are due to minor or major ailments cannot be determined without examinations which are sometimes embarrassing and not entirely painless. First comes the rectal exam carried out by the finger of the physician. Then the cleansing laxatives and enemas are followed by the insertion of barium into the rectum, or you may be asked to bend over a table that is tilted to allow instruments such as colonoscopes to enter and give the doctor a direct view of the lining membrane of the colon.

All these events require time, money, and considerable patience, particularly since the procedures can be unpleasant and sometimes painful. Yet their purpose is to diagnose whether disease exists, and if present, its nature and extent. Appropriate and timely therapy depends upon proper diagnosis, established by a thorough examination of the rectum and colon. The right treatment of colon and rectal disorders often reduces symptoms, halts the progression of illness or reverses it, and may be life-saving. Denial of symptoms and delay in getting help represent understandable but dangerous tactics to forestall the inevitable, dangerous because the procrastination may transform manageable problems to serious and uncontrollable ones. Diseases such as cancer and ulcerative colitis progress no matter how fervently we hope that time alone will take care of things, and diverticulitis can raise complex medical and surgical issues. It's appropriate to take an objective look at each of these three diseases.

Diverticulitis

Imagine an automobile tire containing an inner tube. If such a tire wears down far enough, a small knuckle of the inner tube may pop through and create a soft pea-sized bulge that occupies the defect. This is an example of a hernia, in which a soft tissue snugly enters a structural defect in an overlying casing. In the colon, tiny hernias of this kind are called *diverticula*. One would be called a *diverticulum*. Diverticula form when the inner lining of the colon pops through the muscle layers that encase it. Most diverticula occur in the lower third of the colon and are about the size of a cherry pit. A few to hundreds of diverticula usually exist without any symptoms at all. It is noteworthy that the person already possessing diverticula feels absolutely nothing when a new diverticulum develops. People under the age of thirty generally have no diverticula, but half the Americans over age sixty possess them. Thus diverticula first appear in middle age and increase thereafter.

At first, these small bubbles in the bowel wall are not associated with an actual hole in the bowel and so the contents of the colon remain where they belong. The wall of the bubble is not inflamed by bacteria and the term *diverticulosis* signifies nothing more than the condition or the presence of these diverticula. They are often discovered when a barium-enema examination is carried out for the evaluation of colon disease. As the chalky barium flows up from the rectum to fill the colon, the diverticula fill as well and appear as small white pouches on the outer edge of the large bowel. The cause of diverticulosis is not known, but as discussed in the section on fiber, this condition is very uncommon in Africa and Asia. Not only is diverticulosis considered a feature of life in "developed countries" but many physicians believe that diverticula arise because low-fiber (low-residue) diets leave insufficient bulk to ensure proper motility of the colon. The recent emphasis on increasing the amount of fiber eaten in the diet may well lead to a reduction in the amount of diverticulosis seen in Western countries, but it is too early to tell whether this prediction will come true.

To this point, there is little reason for controversy. We know that the pouches called diverticula do not themselves cause symptoms; yet they are blind sacs and the fecal contents in the mainstream of the colon stagnate in these sacs. At unpredictable times, two events occur in one of these diverticula, and they occur nearly simultaneously: perforation and inflammation. Imagine that a very tiny hole occurs in one of the sacs. Bacteria present in the sac spill through the hole and cause inflammation, with white blood cells going to do battle at the site. The inflammation involves a small part of the lining of the abdomen, the peritoneum. The result is the clinical illness called diverticulitis—pain, usually in the lower left part of the abdomen, with fever, chills, and constipation.

Most experts agree that even in the person with a hundred diverticula, already having diverticul*osis* by definition, the acute perforation-inflammation complication called diverticul*itis* involves one, or at the most two, of these sacs. Disagreement arises as to whether the first event is inflammation, with a tiny perforation the second event; whether the two occur simultaneously; or whether the tiny hole is formed first, with inflammation following. Whichever the sequence, it is clear that infection is part of the process, hence the fever and the usefulness of antibiotics in treatment.

In the same way that self-sealing tires don't go flat when a nail punctures the casing, the damage from diverticulitis is limited by the pronounced swelling of tissues that spares the patient a more serious infection where colon contents escape into the entire abdominal cavity. Therefore, a "mild" episode of diverticulitis is due to the perforation-inflammation of one diverticulum that involves only a small area of the lining peritoneum. The rapid onset of symptoms, such as pain and fever with constipation, usually brings the patient promptly to a physician, who can make the diagnosis with little difficulty. Where other conditions are suspected, a barium enema may be done, but most experts feel that a typical attack of acute diverticulitis should first be allowed to subside before a barium enema is carried out. The treatment of diverticulitis requires a hospital admission for bed rest, plenty of fluids given intravenously, relief of pain, and putting the bowel "to rest" by not allowing the patient to eat anything. Because the condition involves infection, even if a local one, antibiotics are important in therapy and help shorten the illness.

If the diagnosis of diverticulitis is delayed so that antibiotics are not given promptly, or if a large diverticulum ruptures, the infection may spread from a local site through the entire abdomen, and into the bloodstream as well. Even if the rupture seals over as a result of inflammation, the bacteria already present can lead to the formation of an abscess, a complication of diverticulitis that may necessitate surgery.

Quite another matter is the need for surgery during an attack of uncomplicated diverticulitis. Equally skilled surgeons have sharply opposed views about both the need and timing of surgery. The pros and cons of these arguments take up chapters in textbooks, but you are right in adopting the view that if bowel surgery can be avoided, all the better. Even though one's judgment may be weakened by the pain and fever of diverticulitis, the potential risk of surgery as well as the benefits is important to hear. The decision for surgery in diverticulitis should involve the collective judgment of both a skilled surgeon and a nonsurgical physician, usually an internist or a family physician. A hasty decision to operate, if not explained and fully justified, should be viewed with suspicion. Intravenous fluids and high doses of antibiotics may work as well—ask even a trusted surgeon why an operation seems so inevitable. If you're not satisfied with the explanation, you have the right to ask for another opinion.

The reverse is true when the other major complication of diverticulosis arises. Diverticula can *bleed,* and bleed massively, propelling patients into operating rooms with little delay. Bleeding usually occurs from one or more of the blood vessels that happen to herniate into the diverticulum along with the lining of the bowel. The diagnosis of the bleeding diverticulum is easier now than in previous years because of the availability of colonoscopes, long flexible tubes through which an expert can see the entire length of the colon and determine where the bleeding point is. Massive intestinal hemorrhage causing rectal bleeding (not vomiting of blood) is more likely due to a bleeding diverticulum than to colitis, cancer, or injury. Although bleeding may stop by itself, persistence for more than a day or two or a sudden increase in rectal bleeding may require immediate surgery. One bit of good news is that a patient with diverticulosis may develop either the complication of infection or bleeding, but not usually both at the same time.

Most diverticula neither perforate and inflame into diverticulitis, nor do they bleed. Yet half of the American population older than sixty years have diverticulosis. Can we prevent these troublesome complications? A diet high in fiber may be a valuable preventive measure. More fiber or bulk widens the colon and as a result lowers the pressure inside it. Although proof is lacking, it makes sense to advise the person with diverticula to eat more fiber, both to prevent the formation of more diverticula and possibly to prevent the complications of diverticulitis and bleeding. Again, to dispel the confusion in names, divertic*losis* means that these tiny pouches exist and diverticul*itis* means the inflammation of such pouches, usually following a small perforation.

Ulcerative Colitis

The word *colitis* to physicians and patients has as many variations in meaning as does the word *burned*. When you hear that latter word, what goes through your mind? A finger placed too near a toaster? A house fire? Too much sun at the beach? Or, as a social example, some poor soul is "burned" when his just-purchased used car won't start. The word "burned" obviously isn't specific at all. Many such words are used in ordinary conversation in various ways but are often misleading when applied to medical diagnoses. In medicine the term *colitis* is a prime example.

Most people who walk the earth with a diagnosis of "colitis" don't have colitis at all. Colitis means true inflammation of the lining wall (mucosa) of the colon. Yet, in the chapter on apparent colon disease, we describe how often irritable bowel syndrome or irregular bowel action is diagnosed as "mucous" colitis, "spastic" colitis, "functional" colitis, or something else. The mucosa that lines the colon in such patients is entirely normal, yet all too often no physician has looked inside. If a doctor has diagnosed your problem as colitis without a careful examination via a sigmoidoscope or colonoscope, and x-rays with a barium enema, do not accept his diagnosis. You may be better off in the hands of another physician.

A form of colitis truly denoting inflammation of the bowel is that related to *turista* or traveler's diarrhea. In such cases, a bacterium or virus is eaten or drunk, multiplies in the small bowel or colon, causes acute inflammation with cramps, diarrhea, and perhaps fever, and then goes away by itself. *Turista* is a form of colitis, but one due to an identifiable infection that subsides by itself or with appropriate antibiotic therapy. It is therefore clearly different from ulcerative colitis.

The colitis of ulcerative colitis means that inflammation of the mucosa exists, and when inflamed, the colon tries to empty itself with great frequency, thus causing the diarrhea. For blood to appear in the stool as a result of colitis, an ulcer has to break the "skin" of these lining cells. Thus the hallmarks of ulcerative colitis are blood, pus, and sometimes mucus that accompany diarrhea due to inflammation and open sores in the colon wall. The bleeding ulcers in colitis are situated in the colon; this disease is completely different from the bleeding that may complicate an ulcer located in the first few inches of the *small* bowel, the duodenum.

Some patients with ulcerative colitis experience no more than two or three bowel movements a day, without blood. At the other end of the spectrum, severe disease announces its presence by causing a miserable feeling of ill health, frequent bloody bowel movements, high fever, and fairly severe abdominal cramps. The same patient may have mild disease one month and severe symptoms the next, with no clear reason for the waxing and waning apparent to either patient or doctor. Some ulcerative colitis worsens with infection elsewhere, or with stress, emotional turmoil, and other factors about which we are entirely ignorant. As the symptoms are variable, so is the amount of colon involved. Some patients with ulcerative colitis have disease limited to but a few inches of the rectum, whereas in others the entire colon bears the brunt of the illness. In general, the troublesome symptoms increase as more colon is involved.

The cause of ulcerative colitis is unknown. Hundreds of leads toward finding the cause or causes have been explored by scientists for at least fifty years, without success so far. New investigators join in the hunt every year. Some facts are clear. Ulcerative colitis occurs more commonly in Jews than in non-Jews (another enigma) and the disease is found in all Western countries. The affluent are afflicted more often than the impoverished, but again no one knows why. Perhaps this condition also occurs throughout

Asia and the Indian subcontinent, but in those areas the disease is difficult to distinguish from the colon inflammation due to bacteria such as *Shigella.* Heredity may play a part in its cause, as more than one family member can suffer from true ulcerative colitis. The illness typically begins in teenagers or young adults, but the onset may be as late as age sixty. Later in life the diagnosis is somewhat more difficult since other bowel diseases in advancing years may appear to be ulcerative colitis, yet are not. It takes a fair amount of testing and objective judgment on the part of the physician to diagnose bloody diarrhea correctly at any age, but especially in the elderly.

The diagnosis of ulcerative colitis is made by examining the colon through a proctoscope or colonoscope in search of the characteristic tiny ulcers and inflamed mucosa. A biopsy often done at this time will allow a pathologist to confirm the clinical diagnosis. A barium enema is usually carried out to view the rest of the large bowel, to establish the extent of disease, and to provide evidence that another cause of colitis, especially one due to infectious agents, is *not* the cause of the problem. This last possibility also requires the careful examination of stool specimens in a laboratory skilled at finding the few potential culprits in the immense population of bacteria that thrive in the colon. Only after so extensive an evaluation can a definitive diagnosis be made. Ulcerative colitis must be thought of and treated as a lifelong condition since an acute attack may occur after months or years of no symptoms whatever.

The treatment of acute ulcerative colitis usually requires hospital admission. The bowel is "rested" as described for diverticulitis, and doctors prescribe one of a group of specialized drugs called anti-inflammatory agents. These include cortisone or prednisone and the antibiotic sulfadiazine. Anti-inflammatory drugs of the steroid class, of which prednisone is the most widely used form, represent major drugs used to manage a major condition.

Steroids are potent, sometimes life-saving drugs, but side effects include hypertension, obesity, and loss of calcium from bone. The proper treatment of ulcerative colitis is never easy and should be undertaken only by physicians trained in handling this disease. There are important decisions aside from the one on the use of prednisone. Even simple matters pose dilemmas in treatment. For example, diarrhea is so persistent a problem that patients with ulcerative colitis come to know the location of every bathroom between home and work, yet the use of drugs to stop diarrhea is somewhat hazardous. Many experienced doctors strongly feel that improperly treated or untreated patients have the most difficulty with complications of their ulcerative colitis.

The three major complications of ulcerative colitis are perforation of the colon, inflammation unresponsive to therapy that may require surgical removal of the entire colon, and cancer. Cancer of the colon occurs more commonly in the ulcerative-colitis patient than in others, by a factor of five or more, and continues to be a risk even if the underlying colitis has been quiet for years. Most doctors who follow patients with long-standing ulcerative colitis will search for cancer via a yearly barium enema or colonoscope examination. This emphasizes the long-term vigilance necessary for management of patients with ulcerative colitis. For this reason, such patients tend to gather in the waiting rooms of gastroenterologists and not family physicians.

Although the increased risk of cancer leads some patients to wonder if the entire colon should not be removed when ulcerative colitis is first diagnosed, most patients with ulcerative colitis do *not* develop cancer. In fact, half a group of ulcerative-colitis sufferers do not develop any complication mentioned, and live in usual harmony and occasional disharmony with their colon illness. Since the colon is not directly involved in the process of digesting nutrients important to maintain health, the signs of major weight loss and serious illness are absent, though the energy for everyday life may be reduced when diarrhea occurs.

The first cousin of ulcerative colitis is regional ileitis or Crohn's disease. The inflammation in this disease occurs in the region of the ileum in the small bowel and not the colon. Hence, regional ileitis. Crohn's disease (described originally by Drs. Oppenheimer, Ginsburg, and Crohn) is a true bowel inflammation of unknown cause, as is ulcerative colitis, and even "regional" ileitis sometimes spreads to involve the colon as well. Inflammation and ulcers are prominent, as are lumps of inflammatory cells and white blood cells called granuloma. Many gastroenterologists thus speak of "granulomatous ileitis" or "granulomatous colitis," depending on location. The cause of ileitis is unknown and, as with ulcerative colitis, the disease is more common in Jews. Crohn's disease is a more complex disease than ulcerative colitis because it has a tendency to cause scarring of the intestine, with the important complications of obstruction and false channels (fistulas). Since this disease involves the small bowel where digestion takes place, patients with Crohn's disease are often malnourished and lose weight impressively.

In contrast to those with ulcerative colitis, patients with Crohn's disease lose more weight, have more pain, yet suffer less from bloody diarrhea or the risk of cancer. The disease strikes young people, as does ulcerative colitis, but because of the type and location of the pain, the diagnosis of acute appendicitis is sometimes falsely made. Since the ileum and appendix are anatomic neighbors, and the symptoms are so similar, this confusion is understandable. In recent years doctors have learned that typical Crohn's disease may involve the colon only and spare the ileum altogether. These two diseases, Crohn's disease and ulcerative colitis, may therefore be indistinguishable from one another in certain patients.

Many thousands of Americans lead vigorous and productive lives even though they suffer from ulcerative colitis or regional enteritis. Both are lifelong diseases that can be complicated by acute attacks, bleeding or perforation, and the development of abscesses or fistulas in Crohn's disease. Cancer complicates ulcerative colitis yet spares those with ileitis. Both groups of patients require lifelong attention by concerned physicians.

Precisely the opposite is true for those with apparent colon disease, who are best advised to ignore or deflect symptoms and get on with daily life. The term "colitis" must not be haphazardly invoked to explain any diarrhea or pain or change in bowel habit that defies more precise diagnosis. For every person with three loose bowel movements a day whose supposed "functional" or apparent colon disease is really undiagnosed ulcerative colitis, ten or twenty people lead worried lives because they have been told that they have colitis without the true diagnosis having been established at all. Chapter 3, Apparent Colon Disease, discusses this perplexing issue in greater detail.

Cancer of the Colon

The reason it is so vital to diagnose colon cancer early is that early detection can save lives. Malignant growths in this organ are among the most common and curable of all cancers, if diagnosis leads to proper therapy before the cancer spreads to lymph glands or the liver. Who, then, is responsible for ensuring that a cancer of the large bowel is detected early enough to allow effective treatment? The answer to this is clear—*detection, as always, begins with the patient.* When that patient comes into contact with a doctor, they both participate—the patient presents information and the doctor assesses it. The "clinical history" of illness is therefore the product of a genuine patient-physician relationship.

The single impediment to the early diagnosis of colon cancer is the reticence of patients to discuss their bowel habits, presumably because the truly innocent goings-on in our bowels are considered rather sinister secrets. Somewhere near the end of Queen Victoria's reign or the beginning of Freudian psychotherapy, the Western world collectively decided that bowel function, and all substances reminding us of it, were entirely repellent and unworthy of civilized conversation. The legacies of these beliefs have been twofold, the first of which is that many swear words and nasty oaths in Western languages are scatological in content.

The second, far more serious, is that the failure to discuss bowel action delays the diagnosis of colon cancer. It is understandable that people do not freely converse about bowel movements with their friends, but the reluctance to do so with their physicians is the final manifestation of our continuing aversion for the subject. As a result, the change in bowel habits that often signifies the existence of bowel cancer remains unmentioned in the examining room, and thus a valuable opportunity to uncover an early malignancy is lost. So our first message must not be forgotten: *discuss changes in bowel activity with your physician.* No doctor is embarrassed by talking over these matters, and so the natural hesitancy of the patient must be overcome if he or she is going to be properly cared for from a gastrointestinal point of view. If your doctor is too busy to listen to you, find another. On the other hand, if your visits to the doctor always concern your bowel problem, you likely possess a normal colon.

Cancers of the colon and rectum are unusual before the age of thirty-five, but thereafter the incidence steadily increases with each passing year, only to wane again in persons over age seventy. The cause of bowel cancer is unknown despite its high incidence, but some clues have recently surfaced that eventually may yield better understanding as to how these tumors arise. For example, colon cancer remains a genuinely rare occurrence in those countries where high-fiber diets rich in indigestible bulk are consumed, as in most countries in Africa. Conversely, high rates of bowel cancer are found in countries where citizens eat a diet highly refined in order to remove bulk, as is the case in the United States. Where beef and other animal meats are consumed in large quantities, colon cancer is common.

Japan was a nation whose citizens were spared colon cancer until more Western-type fast-food products such as hamburgers were introduced, and the growing popularity of such food in Japan has coincided with startling increases in malignant growths in the large bowel. Numerous medical scientists in Japan are intensely seeking the reason for this association. There is some evidence that the bacteria living quietly in the colon can convert otherwise harmless environmental or food chemicals into cancer-causing agents that then languish in the lower bowel and harm the cells of the colon. Theories such as this one are currently unproven, but the marked differences in incidence of colon cancer among citizens of various countries are easy to verify and in many ways suggest strongly that what we eat may influence cancer development. A number of thoughtful gastroenterologists now believe that if Americans eat less meat and more fiber, the rate of cancer of the colon will begin to decline. Proof is still years away.

Only two symptoms of colon cancer are worth discussing in any detail, and everyone should be aware of them. The first is abdominal pain with or without the aforementioned change in bowel habits. Aunt Millie, whose medicine chest is stuffed with laxatives to cope with lifelong constipation, develops either diarrhea or simply cramps with her usual infrequent movement—*that* is a change in bowel habits. Or Grandpa, whose bowel he describes as "dependable as a Swiss watch ever since the Great Depression," has a few weeks of loose stools that won't tighten up—*that* is also a change in bowel habits. Stools that look like pencils but used to look like sausages—*that's* a change, too. Ninety-nine of a hundred such people will *not* have cancer, but one of them will. So the arithmetic has it that if 30,000 people talk about their recent bowel symptoms with doctors who are carefully listening to them, 300 cancers will be detected. And it is a sobering fact that about 300 colon cancers are detected *daily* in the United States.

The second important symptom of bowel cancer is the loss of blood. If you describe it, it's a symptom. The doctor finds signs. If you notice blood, a cupful in the toilet bowl or merely a red streak in the stool, that is all you have to see to let yourself know that something suspicious is going on. If you ignore this symptom you do so at your own peril. As mentioned before, red blood should never be ascribed to hemorrhoids or other lesser diseases of the bowel, and must be regarded with concern. Unless iron tablets have blackened your stool, black means bleeding from the *small* bowel, as occurs with duodenal ulcers. To delay getting medical help even for twenty-four hours when black stools occur is to roll dice with your health— and perhaps your life.

A third way that bleeding may occur is in the form of blood loss so slow that the person does not see anything red in the bowl or black or red in the stool; this is because a few drops here and there simply get lost within the brown mass. Anemia follows from the loss of iron in these crimson drops, and anemia will make patients tired, listless, and pale. Because many colon cancers bleed secretly in this way, an annual checkup should include not only a rectal examination with the doctor's finger skillfully exploring the lower few inches of the bowel but also a chemical test of the retrieved stool for occult blood; this is so easy to do that it should never be neglected. If you see blood, or if you feel tired and people say you look pale, make a hasty visit to your physician and while there pay attention to what the doctor is doing and attempt to see to it that the examination is complete. Every day patients are given iron tablets to correct anemia, and the blood count improves; the tragedy in some of these people is that the anemia is itself but a sign of the slowly bleeding and growing colon cancer.

Once you're in the office the doctor will ask you about bowel habits, but if he or she does not it is your responsibility to volunteer information on any changes that have occurred, including the suspicion of bleeding from the bowel. A good doctor will then examine the rectum, test a stool smear for occult blood, schedule a proctoscopy (to look into your rectum through a rigid, thin tube) and possibly recommend a barium-enema x-ray examination. Only a few colon cancers will escape detection by these four maneuvers, so if nothing is found, as is usually the case, you can rest assured that a tumor is very unlikely to be present. Sometimes all these tests needn't be done when your symptoms have just started; the decision to hold off is often justified and depends on how concerned your physician is about the possibility of cancer. Under certain circumstances it is best to wait and see what develops, but frequent stool tests for blood are easy to do and important while the waiting goes on.

The message for you, the patient, is this: If you or your doctor ignores the subtle signs of colon cancer, the loss of time will allow the tumor to advance to an untreatable stage. Once the proper diagnosis is made and prompt surgery takes place, your chance of living five years after the detection of colon cancer is presently about 50 percent in the United States. As cancer survival goes, this figure is encouraging. However, if the cancer has spread to even a single lymph node, then the five-year survival rate drops to 20 percent. The surgery for colon cancer *may* leave the patient with a colostomy in which feces empty through a surgically created hole in the abdominal wall and pass into a baglike appliance. This sounds unpleasant, but most people adapt to the inconvenience with amazing ease, and concern over having a colostomy quickly subsides. In addition, "colostomy clubs" in most cities allow patients to share experiences and support each other through rough times. The American Cancer Society has abundant information to help you.

Several years ago a flurry of excitement followed reports that a test of the blood could be used to diagnose cancer of the colon. These tests measure the blood level of a cancer product whose initials are CEA, and the use of this test has become widespread in the United States and other countries. Unfortunately, CEA testing has so far not been proven valuable in the detection of very early colon malignancies and has for this reason not made a significant impact on the statistics of colon cancer survival. An extensive research program is currently under way to improve the testing of the blood for the existence of clues to colon and other cancers.

Polyps

Finally, we address the problem of polyps in the colon. Polyps are tumors on the lining of the large bowel or rectum—some are malignant and others are benign, and they can vary in size from a pinhead to a golf ball. Although many polyps have stalks or stems that give them the appearance of mushrooms, others are stuck firmly up against the colon lining. Regardless of their shape, these polyps reveal their presence either by bleeding in a manner similar to that of colon cancer, or are detected by chance during examination of the bowel by x-ray or proctoscopy. It is not uncommon to find more than one polyp in a patient; some have ten or twenty present at once.

If one or more polyps are detected, your doctor is immediately confronted by the question of what to do. Big polyps, especially the ones that are not on stalks, may harbor malignant cells. The decision to remove most polyps has recently become easier because of the technical advance of colonoscopy. The colonoscope, an ominous-looking but thin and flexible tube, is passed through the rectum far into the bowel so that the polyps can be located by direct vision. Once found, polyps are snipped off by an ingenious electrical-metallic snare that simultaneously cuts the polyp loose and prevents bleeding by heating shut the blood vessel that entered the fleshy lump. Polyps removed in this way are usually retrieved and examined micro-scopically to determine whether or not they harbor cancer cells.

The entire issue of whether polyp formation is itself related to the development of later colon cancer is a con-troversial one not fully settled at this time. Cynics claim that the removal of polyps is a maneuver to improve the physician's financial health rather than the medical health of the patient. However, the advance of colonoscopy has allowed the removal of polyps without the hazards and discomfort of operations that involve entering the abdomi-nal cavity directly, and large polyps may contain malig-nant cells. Colon cancers themselves are never treated by colonoscopy as they call for removal of a large portion of the bowel.

In summary, colon cancer and, to a lesser extent, co-lon polyps announce themselves as changes in bowel habits with or without bleeding, and the bleeding that occurs may be unnoticed by the patient until iron loss causes ane-mia. The detection of colon tumors is an enterprise which combines the observations of the patient and the careful appraisal of symptoms and signs by the patient's physi-cian. Thus both individuals are involved in the important task of *early* detection of colon cancer before these tumors advance to an untreatable state. The somber statistics on mortality due to colon cancer nowadays may improve with research into the cause of these tumors, but until more information is available *early detection* is the key to long survival.

9
Afterword

As a physician, I am constantly reminded how seriously people take the matter of their bowels. By "bowels" I mean the colon and its product—feces—and not the rest of the gastrointestinal tract, where the whole process of digestion takes place. It is the bowel habit and especially its variations that seem so important. What other explanation for the middle-aged man whose heart attack occurred three days ago, now worried not about his life or his family, his finances or his job, but rather that he has not moved his bowels since he was brought to the hospital? Millions care passionately about bowel function. Because the subjects in this book have been treated frankly, not buried in detailed descriptions of digestion, we may be faulted for having dared to invade the one area of personal geography that should remain unexplored. Many other once-private subjects have come into the open. Yet, until now, only a few volumes about the colon and its product have appeared.

I confess to not knowing why. Is it the way we are brought up? Growing out of infancy is marked by three episodes: the first word, the first unaided step, and the first formed stool that thuds into the potty seat. A sophisticated and open-minded woman recently recalled a dinner party she herself interrupted to lead the young couples from the dining table to the bathroom to view the accomplishment of her first-born. Perhaps success at toilet training marks the end of infancy, and in later life, unless you want to be considered infantile, you should not mention the subject outside the office of your private physician. Other valid explanations can be offered for the suppression of talk about the bowels, but none come to mind. Is such talk crude and uncivilized to the listener's ear?

As a child "the bowels" seemed no more important to me than did the teeth or fingernails; and no one talked to me about the bowels, nor to each other about them. Yet, when radio news was interrupted by advertisements for Carter's Little Liver Pills, the abrupt and tense silence of the adults around the table struck me as peculiar and mysterious. This silence was sometimes followed by a certain look, at least where I grew up. It was a momentary but intense gridlock of eyes nowadays reserved for liaisons or important secrets. On a related subject, the noisy explosion of gas that unexpectedly escaped from someone young or old caused suppressed giggles in children, and a glacial vacant silence of elders so strange that only a brave fool would have questioned it. My own son at age four unashamedly showed us the "poop dots" in his underwear and occasionally waved his stools farewell before flushing. I hope my parental pride at his naturalness is not misplaced.

Yet how clearly I remember my grandfather Max, not at the dinner table but on the can, his face cheery and round. Max loved many things in life: his profession of medicine, the symphony, books, his children, and his cigars. In most things he was an intensely rational man and he commented once that he smoked cigars only to accompany important engagements, while listening to music or discussing medicine or digesting a good supper, among friends. He stopped talking there, but my memory races on faithfully to what I recall from the very next morning—"Opa" Max sitting on the can on a cold January morning in our upstairs bathroom with his pants down and the bathroom door not quite shut, his cigar lit, and his mustachioed pink face expectant. Half smiling and pleased at the act, he passed a fragrant stool and inspected the product with the calm and scientific thoroughness of a physician who knows the importance of what he's doing.

I was about six years old when I saw this, but it was apparent that if Opa cared enough about defecation to smoke cigars while doing it, with that look on his face—it had to be big-time stuff! To take the matter to the edge of propriety, how often will a parent call through a closed bathroom door, "Are you done in there?" Within a year or two, as a child enters adolescence, the call may change to "What are you doing in there?" Accept it or not, the act of defecation and sexual impulses and feelings are linked in various and complex ways. No doubt a variety of opinions can be found on this subject, as can speculations on the phenomenon of reading before, during, or after the act of moving the bowels. Perhaps the next book on the bowels should be written by a psychiatrist.

Until the subject was discussed in medical school, I believed as do others that food falls into the stomach and gets digested and then drops into the rectum and turns brown and knocks and emerges. My childhood friends shared the belief that the "bowels" served primarily to manufacture tomorrow's bowel movement. In college I was instructed that the stomach lies near the top and may cause bloating or heartburn, but mankind pays more attention to the bottom. And now I've learned that moving the bowels remains the single inviolable reason for missing any other appointment, including the most urgent phone call. It's truly uncivilized to deny the validity of that excuse. Why? And why is it that the business of the bowel so bothers people?

Few preoccupations increase with age as does that with our bowels. As a young doctor I learned how to ask questions and listen carefully to patients' answers, the oldest and still the best technique for diagnosing disease. For obvious reasons, sick and frightened people have little patience for the never-ending stream of questions from the doctor. There is one exception, illustrated in an exchange recorded with an old lady from a nursing home, admitted to the hospital with a broken hip. Other possible problems, body system by system, had to be explored by the physician.

"Appetite all right?"

"Fair."

"Any foods bother you?"

"No."

"Any pain in your abdomen after you eat?"

"No."

"Ever had yellow jaundice?"

"No."

"Any surgery on your stomach?"

"No."

"Any bleeding from down below?"

"Down below?" The old lady releases a withering stare.

"Your vagina, I meant."

"No. Of course not."

"You went through the menopause then?"

"Before you were born, sonny."

A pause to regroup. "All right. Any shortness of breath?"

"No." She now turns painfully from this rapid-fire interrogation.

"Chest pain?"

Pause. "No."

"Any trouble with your urine?"

"Not lately."

"How about your bowels?"

She turns back. A smile! "No, doctor, thank you, they're fine, but I do so appreciate your asking."

On a few occasions a bowel movement really deserves the attention paid to it. The first call following hemorrhoid surgery may be vividly remembered for life. After the delivery of a child, the pain of defecation intensifies the fear that the episiotomy stitches will break. Then there's the first formed stool—hallelujah!—after uncounted Lomotil tablets and the runs in Mexico. And the prayerful thanks upon passing the first normal stool after treatment for ulcerative colitis, cancer, diverticulitis, or simply breaking the laxative habit. No doubt every reader can recall one of these or a similarly meaningful event.

Most of the time we look at what we have just passed, not only because it is something that emerges from us, available for inspection on an almost daily basis, but because it has come from deep within and so ought to be important. Sometimes it is crucial. Any rectal bleeding requires prompt and thorough evaluation. Almost every other long-lasting variation in bowel habit, unless accompanied by severe pain, high fever, or weight loss, is hardly worth worrying about. This book should be considered successful if you can now discard the idea that one, only one, but definitely one bowel movement per day is the appropriate bowel habit. Deviating from some hypothetical "normal" need not propel you to a physician to find out why. Yet, if something does go wrong with your colon, get help promptly and keep in mind that you have a right to good health care. Many good doctors learn a great deal through questioning you, by carefully examining the abdomen from the outside, and by performing a rectal examination as well as one on the stool to see if blood is present. With the few special exceptions noted in this book, most bowel complaints, from gas to hemorrhoids to traveler's diarrhea to "irregularity," are no more important to the health of humankind than is another gray hair.

If the information in this book helps you feel better about this most private of personal concerns, we have been successful. Just imagine. When every new bit of information seems to add to the anxiety of life—what can and does go wrong, and how unexpected and permanent such bad news can be—it must feel good to know that nearly all irregular bowel habits and new symptoms are no more worrisome than a few days of the blues. This is the reassuring message that doctors are giving patients today as yesterday, and some of those patients have complaints of gas, hemorrhoids, alternating periods of constipation and diarrhea, or merely concern that, as a patient once confided to me, "A day without stool is a day without sunshine."

Often the reassurance succeeds when the message follows a long, expensive, and rather unpleasant "workup" by a medical specialist; and we repeat for the last time that sudden pain, rectal bleeding, or a change in your bowel habit in midlife or thereafter requires prompt evaluation. Most people have bowel complaints that are *not* the worrisome ones listed, and for you who have learned from this book how your bowel works, why symptoms occur, and what you can do about them, you probably feel better about the health of your colon and your body in general. We share your good feeling.

Index